AF616132

ALLERGIES AND INFECTIOUS DISEASES

SEPSIS

DIAGNOSIS, MANAGEMENT AND HEALTH OUTCOMES

ALLERGIES AND INFECTIOUS DISEASES

Additional books in this series can be found on Nova's website under the Series tab.

Additional e-books in this series can be found on Nova's website under the e-book tab.

ALLERGIES AND INFECTIOUS DISEASES

SEPSIS

DIAGNOSIS, MANAGEMENT AND HEALTH OUTCOMES

NANCY KHARDORI, M.D., PH.D.
EDITOR

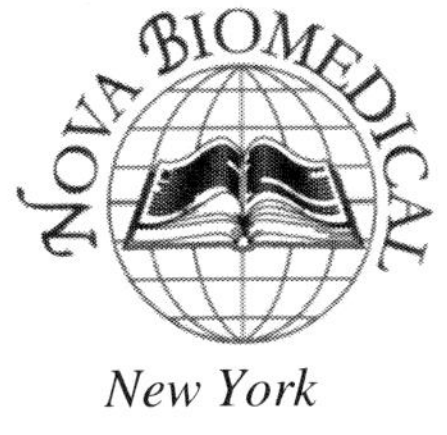

New York

For permission to use material from this book please contact us:
Telephone 631-231-7269; Fax 631-231-8175
Web Site: http://www.novapublishers.com

Additional color graphics may be available in the e-book version of this book.

Library of Congress Cataloging-in-Publication Data

ISBN: 978-1-63117-244-1

Library of Congress Control Number: 2014930680

Published by Nova Science Publishers, Inc. † New York

Contents

Preface

The late 19th and early 20th century saw a rapid development in the diagnosis and management of diseases caused by infectious agents. In vitro cultivation of bacteria made specific diagnosis of bacterial diseases and testing of antibacterial agents possible. Subsequent availability of a number of antibacterial agents and vaccines against childhood viral diseases made a remarkable impact on the morbidity and mortality associated with infectious diseases especially in the developed countries with a strong public health infrastructure.

However, the continued advances in critical care and antimicrobial therapy have failed to make an impact on the morbidity and mortality associated with sepsis syndrome. The insensitivity of the current culture based diagnostics is a significant contributing factor as is the ongoing development of resistance to antibacterial agents. However, the critical role in the pathogenesis of sepsis syndrome is played by a very complex and intricate interaction between the infecting agent and the host biological and immunological systems. The outcome is unpredictable and very well described by the quote "I suspect that the host is caught up in mistaken inappropriate and unquestionably self-destructive mechanisms by the very multiplicity of defenses available to him, defenses which to not seem to have been designed to operate in net coordination with each other. The end result is not defense; it is an agitated, committee-directed, harum-scarum effort to make war." Lewis Thomas.

The goal of this book on Sepsis syndrome is to provide the state of the art knowledge in an area which is under extensive investigation. The first chapter provides a thorough review of pathogenesis at the cellular and molecular levels. This followed by the two chapters on myocardial dysfunction and acute kidney injury, two of the major organs involved in multiorgan failure and poor outcomes in sepsis syndrome. The authors describe the currently available modalities of treatment as well as some of the promising and novel agents with the potential of improving outcomes in sepsis. The Chapters four and five discuss the epidemiology and management of sepsis syndrome in neonates and adults respectively. The impact of gestational age in neonates and co-morbidities in the elderly on the incidence and outcomes of sepsis syndrome are well described. The contribution of preventable factors is described in Chapter 6 along with a detailed description of the recommendations offered by the "surviving sepsis campaign". Given the extensive use of medical devices especially in critically and chronically ill patients and their association with sepsis syndrome, an independent Chapter 7 is devoted to this subject. The Chapter 8 describes the shortcomings of the current methods available for diagnosis of sepsis syndrome and the potential of upcoming and investigational diagnostics with a focus on non-culture based technologies like biomarkers and genomics. The control of the common metabolic disorder of hyperglycemia and diabetes mellitus has been shown to have a positive impact on the outcomes of sepsis syndrome. The last chapter in this book offers a detailed discussion on the intricacies of glycemic control in sepsis syndrome.

One of the major strengths of this book is the ensemble of the authors relating experiences from various continents of the world on epidemiological, clinical and basic sciences. It is our expectation that the book will be of value to a variety of readers including medical students, basic scientists and clinicians.

I owe personal gratitude to Brenda J. Walden, BS for her technical assistance in getting this volume ready for publication.

Nancy Khardori, M.D, Ph.D.
Professor, Division of Infectious Diseases
Department of Internal Medicine and
Department of Microbiology
and Molecular Cell Biology
Eastern Virginia Medical School
Norfolk, Virginia, USA.

In: Sepsis
Editor: Nancy Khardori

ISBN: 978-1-63117-244-1

Chapter 1

Sepsis: Molecular Events, Interventions and Novel Approaches

Markus Bosmann, M.D.[1,2] ***and Peter A. Ward, M.D.***[3*]

[1]Center for Thrombosis and Hemostasis,
University Medical Center, Mainz, Germany
[2]Department of Hematology and Oncology,
University Medical Center, Mainz, Germany
[3]Department of Pathology, University of Michigan Medical School,
Ann Arbor, MI US

Abstract

Sepsis is defined as a systemic inflammatory response syndrome caused by infectious pathogens. Sepsis is a life-threatening disease ultimately leading to multi-organ failure and often death. It is estimated that worldwide more than 3 million cases of sepsis occur annually with mortality rates around 20-50%, increasing with age. During the past decades a great number of interventional pharmacologic trials in humans failed to demonstrate efficacy in reversing the unfavorable course of sepsis. The development and progression of sepsis is characterized by spreading of a formerly localized infection, typically involving bacteria, fungi or viruses. In addition to the release of microbial toxins, an inadequate immune response contributes to organ dysfunction during sepsis. Activation of the complement system generates large amounts of the highly reactive complement anaphylatoxin, C5a. Innate and adaptive immune cells are activated, resulting in production of reactive oxygen species, cytokines/chemokines as well as triggering the appearance of neutrophil-extracellular traps and extracellular histones. During various phases of human sepsis a considerable degree of immunosuppression caused by apoptosis of lymphocytes often develops. Novel treatment approaches will be necessary to exploit the recent advances in understanding of the molecular events during sepsis.

[*] Corresponding author: Peter A. Ward, MD, University of Michigan Medical School, Department of Pathology, 1301 Catherine Road, Ann Arbor, MI 48109-5602.

List of Abbreviations

APC	activated protein C
CLP	cecal ligation and puncture
C5a	complement component C5a
C5aR	C5a receptor 1, CD88
C5L2	C5a receptor 2, GPR77
EBI3	Epstein Barr virus induced gene 3
HMGB1	high mobility group protein B 1
IL-27	interleukin-27
LPS	lipopolysaccharide (bacterial)
MAPK	mitogen-activated protein kinase
MODS	multiple-organ dysfunction syndrome
NETs	neutrophil extracellular traps
PD-1	programmed cell death protein 1
PD-1L	programmed cell death protein 1 ligand
PI3K	phosphatidylinositide 3-kinase
PMNs	polymorphonuclear neutrophils
ROS	reactive oxygen species
SIRS	systemic inflammatory response syndrome
TNFα	tumor necrosis factor alpha

Introduction

Sepsis is a life-threatening disease and was first described in ancient medical literature more than 2000 years ago. The term "sepsis" is derived from the old Greek word "σῆψις" describing a condition of putrefaction and decay. It is now clear that sepsis is a complication of severe infections with pathogenic microorganisms. The current guidelines for the diagnosis of sepsis include several clinical criteria: hypo-/hyperthermia, hypotension, tachycardia, tachypnea and altered mental status. Clinical pathology testing is typically conspicuous for parameters of infection such as leukocytosis/leukopenia, elevated C-reactive protein and increased procalcitonin concentrations in blood.

Septic shock refers to a sepsis-induced reduction in systemic vascular resistance leading to hypotension that is resistant to fluid resuscitation. Severe sepsis develops because of tissue hypoperfusion, resulting in subsequent organ dysfunction. Such complications of sepsis include acute renal injury, acute lung injury with respiratory insufficiency, septic cardiomyopathy, acute liver injury and abnormal blood coagulation (consumptive coagulopathy).

Progression of sepsis to multiple-organ dysfunction syndrome (MODS) and multiple organ failure is often associated with a lethal outcome. The systemic inflammatory response syndrome (SIRS) has similar clinical features as sepsis but typically occurs in the absence of infection. SIRS is a sepsis-like syndrome in response to a non-infectious insults such as trauma, burns, hemorrhagic shock, pancreatitis, vasculitis and autoimmune disorders.

Epidemiologic studies have estimated an incidence of more than 2,800,000 annual cases of sepsis in high-income countries worldwide. [1] Over the past decades in the United States there was an annualized increase in the occurrence of sepsis of 8.7% each year to more than 600,000 cases. [2] This increase in the incidence of sepsis is most likely due to a higher prevalence of risk factors in population. Recognized risk factors for the development of sepsis are immunosuppression, advanced aged (≥65 years), diabetes and cancer. Advances in critical care medicine have led to a decrease in mortality rates, ranging from 20-50%. The high variations in the estimated mortality rates found in the literature may be explained by variations in inclusion criteria of patient cohorts (sepsis, severe sepsis, septic shock). To date, sepsis due to gram-positive bacterial infection is more common as compared to gram-negative bacterial pathogens. [2] While the numbers of sepsis caused by fungal pathogens has clearly increased over the past decades, only a few viral pathogens have been confirmed to precipitate septic shock.

Pathophysiologic Considerations

Inflammation is a major hallmark in the development and progression of severe sepsis and septic shock. Clinically, inflammation is described by five classical signs: redness, swelling, pain, heat and disturbances in function. In detail, microorganisms or non-infectious insults trigger acute inflammation, which involves regulation of local blood vessel permeability, generation of inflammatory mediators and recruitment of immune cells to the site of inflammation.

Increased blood vessel permeability promotes the influx of plasma proteins to the extracellular compartment. This includes microbe-binding proteins (mannose-binding-lectin, C-reactive protein, antibodies), precursors of peptide mediators (complement factors, high-molecular weight kininogen) and coagulation factors. Local resident immune cells (tissue macrophages, mast cells), connective tissue cells and local parenchymal cells may all participate in the very early phases of inflammation.

These cells release a wide spectrum of substances such as defensins, lipid mediators, histamine, cytokines and chemokines. These mediators trigger a chemotactic wave of invading polymorphonuclear neutrophils (PMNs) entering the site of inflammation from the blood stream within a few hours. PMNs combat microorganisms by phagocytosis, release of their toxic granules and respiratory burst/reactive oxygen species (ROS) and nitric oxide. During the later phases of inflammation bridging of innate immune defenses towards adaptive immunity involves migration, selection and proliferation of specific T cells and B cells for mounting antigen-specific defense mechanisms. While inflammation aims to eliminate pathogens and recovery from toxic insults, the immune responses themselves can also promote tissue injury. For example, ROS and cytotoxic proteins released from intracellular granules of immune cells not only kill bacteria and fungi but can also damage host bystander cells. In addition, cytotoxic NKT cells and T cells can initiate apoptosis of virus infected cells via perforin-dependent mechanisms.

One central question of sepsis research is "*What goes wrong with the immune responses in sepsis?*" There is little disagreement that dysregulated host immune responses can progress to a lethal sepsis-like syndrome (SIRS) even in the absence of a pathogenic microorganism.

A critical event in sepsis is the failure to confine infection to a localized area. Generally, it is considered an adverse event when microorganisms invade the blood circulation. For example, activation of coagulation during inflammation may seal off an area of infection. Solid fibrin networks may contribute to abscess formation, which is frequently observed during gram-positive infection.

Transient small numbers of bacteria in circulation can also occur in healthy individuals and are cleared by the phagocytic system in spleen and liver. In this process platelets may associate with Kupffer cells in the liver while encountering bacteremia.[3] However, many of the underlying mechanisms that determine the failure to prevent systemic spread of infection are incompletely understood. During the early phases of sepsis a state of exuberant immune activation occurs ("hyperinflammation"; see Figure 1).

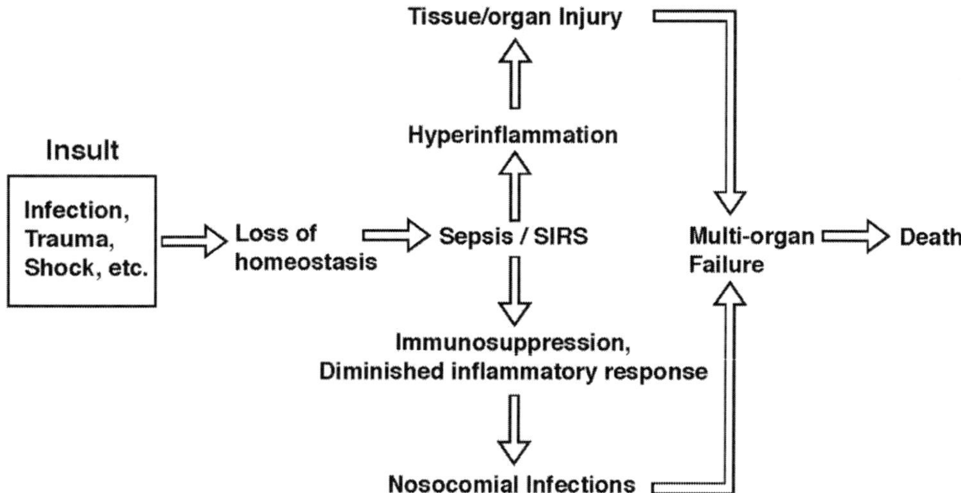

Figure 1. Immunoregulation during Sepsis. Insults by infectious microorganisms, trauma, shock, etc. disturb organ homeostasis and may progress to sepsis/SIRS. Unbalanced inflammation can manifest as either a tissue destructive, hyperinflammatory syndrome as an early event or, at later stages of sepsis, result in profound and persistent immunosuppression and hypoinflammation, both of which render the host susceptible to additional opportunistic infections.

For example, many proinflammatory mediators such as TNFα, IL-6 and IL-1β are released into circulation. When such purified mediators are injected into healthy research animals, sepsis-like symptoms (fever, hypotension, tachycardia) ensue. On the other side, the later stages of sepsis are characterized by profound immunosuppression ("hypo-inflammation"). Lymphocyte apoptosis, necrosis of innate immune cells at the site of bacterial encounter, cytokine-mediated suppression of inflammation and inadequate emergency hematopoiesis decrease the ability of the immune system to effectively fight remaining microorganisms. A better insight into the pathogenesis of sepsis seems mandatory for beneficial therapeutic interventions in the future.

The passages below highlight several critical molecular events as currently understood in sepsis. An overview of several potential targets for pharmacological interventions in sepsis is shown in Table 1.

Table 1. Novel Molecular targets for potential therapeutic interventions in sepsis

Interventions in sepsis with lack of efficacy in clinical trials		
Target	***Therapeutic Strategy***	***References***
Activated human protein C signaling	Recombinant drotrecogin alpha	[50]
Tumor necrosis factor alpha	Neutralizing antibody	[49]
Lipopolysaccharides	Neutralizing antibody	[51]
Interleukin-1 receptor antagonist	Recombinant IL-1Ra	[52, 53]
Eicosanoids	Small molecule inhibitors	[54, 55]
Nitric oxide	Small molecule inhibitors	[56]
Reactive oxygen species	Antioxidants	[57]
Potential interventions in sepsis with no or pending clinical trials		
Target	***Therapeutic Strategy***	***References***
C5a / C5aR / C5L2	Neutralizing antibody	[12, 17]
Extracellular histones	Neutralizing antibody, Enzymatic cleavage	[29]
Interleukin-27	Neutralizing antibody	[18]
Interleukin-7	Recombinant IL-7	[41, 42]
Programmed cell death protein 1	Neutralizing antibody	[43, 44]
High mobility group B1 protein	Neutralizing antibody, recombinant HMGB1 A box	[33]
Vagus nerve stimulation	Electric devices (implantable or transcutaneous)	[9]

Molecular Events and Novel Interventions in Sepsis

The cholinergic anti-inflammatory pathway (CAIP)

Communication between the immune system and the central nervous system utilizes the sympathetic and parasympathetic nerves. [4, 5] For instance, the central nervous system senses inflammation by afferent vagal nerves. The vagal nerve is also the major efferent neuronal conductor to internal organs including the heart, liver, small intestine and spleen. Sequences of action potentials trigger the release of neuronal messenger molecules at the site of vagal nerve endings in the spleen. These messengers stimulate a memory phenotype population of T cells to produce acetylcholine. [6] Acetyl choline is a major parasympathetic transmitter and a major factor of the "inflammatory reflex" for controlling lymphocytes and macrophages in the spleen. These cholinergic mechanisms primarily suppress inflammation. Acetylcholine signaling is dependent on the presence of the α7 nicotinic acetylcholine receptor (α7nAChR) on macrophages and lymphocytes. For example, acetylcholine regulates ATP-induced Ca^{2+} currents in macrophages via α7nAChR. [7] Vagotomy results in increased cytokine production, leukocyte chemotaxis, liver damage and lower survival in experimental sepsis. [8, 9] Artificial vagus nerve stimulation by transcutaneous or implantable electrical devices has anti-inflammatory effects and may be a potential therapeutic intervention in sepsis.

Complement Component C5a

The complement system aims to eliminate pathogens by means of opsonization, direct pathogen lysis and chemotaxis/regulation of immune cells. [10] Molecular patterns of extracellular microorganisms are recognized by preformed antibodies (classical pathway), mannose-binding lectin/ficolins (lectin pathway) or spontaneous hydrolysis of C3 on any foreign surface devoid of host complement inhibitory factors (alternative pathway). All three pathways of complement activation generate the anaphylactic complement cleavage products, C3a, C4a and C5a. These anaphylatoxins promote inflammation by increasing leukocyte chemotaxis, blood vessel permeability and degranulation of endothelial cells and immune cells. The specific biological potency ranks C5a over the other anaphylatoxins (C5a>C3a>C4a). As a safeguard to prevent toxic effects of C5a, rapid clearance mechanisms for C5a operate under normal circumstances. After entering the blood circulation C5a is enzymatically cleaved by carboxypeptidases within minutes into less active $C5a_{desArg}$. In addition, uptake into spleen and kidneys provides final removal of C5a from the blood stream. C5a and $C5a_{desArg}$ are ligands for two homologous G-protein coupled seven-transmembrane-spanning receptors. [11] The C5aR receptor (CD88, C5aR1) is abundantly expressed on myeloid cells (PMNs, macrophages) and in lower numbers also on lymphocytes and non-immune cells. Binding of C5a and $C5a_{desArg}$ to C5aR initiates rapid intracellular Ca^{2+} transients for promotion of chemotaxis. C5aR also activates PI3K/Akt and MAPK signaling pathways for regulation of transcriptional activation of genes with immune functions. The role of the second C5a receptor, C5L2 (GPR77, C5aR2), remains somewhat enigmatic. C5L2 is also expressed by phagocytic cells, does not trigger $Ca2^{+}$ transients but may modulate PI3K/Akt and MAPK signaling in PMNs.

In severe sepsis exuberant quantities of C5a are generated by massive complement activation. The normal range of C5 concentrations in plasma are 55-115 µg/ml. Enzymatic conversion of all C5 in plasma would theoretically result in concentrations of C5a around 5 µg/ml. Detectable levels of C5a in plasma of patients with severe sepsis can be 0.1 µg/ml and sometimes approach 1 µg/ml. However, taking into account the short half-life of C5a in circulation, measurements of C5a at single time points are not necessarily representative for the total amounts of released C5a. Therefore the biological effects of C5a during sepsis are better assessed by the use of C5a neutralizing antibodies or the experimental use of transgenic mice with deficiency of either C5aR or C5L2.

Blocking of C5a using neutralizing antibodies in polymicrobial sepsis (induced by the ligation and puncture procedure; CLP) improves survival rates and reduces bacteremia in rodents. 12] Exuberant release of C5a during sepsis most likely results in saturation of C5a binding sites on leukocytes. While gene expression of C5aR is up-regulated on leukocytes and non-immune cells during sepsis, C5a ligation with C5aR also triggers receptor internalization. A paradoxal shut-down of crucial functions of PMNs can occur, which includes reduced phagocytic activity, diminished production of ROS and impaired release of toxic granule products. In tissue macrophages, C5a in high concentrations can suppress macrophage functions and LPS/TLR4-induced production of proinflammatory cytokines via induction of IL-10 release. [13] On the other hand, C5a promotes the release of TNFα and IL-6 which can have adverse effects during sepsis. In endothelial cells C5a positively regulates chemokine release (e.g., IL-8) and pro-thrombotic tissue factor. Consumptive coagulopathy is often seen in severe sepsis and considered a bad omen. Blockade of C5a by neutralizing antibodies reduces the degree of abnormalities in the coagulation and fibrinolytic cascades. [14]

C5a contributes to the development of septic cardiomyopathy most likely by direct binding to C5aR on cardiomyocytes. Consecutively, C5a modulates changes in the production of inflammatory mediators as well as the electrophysiology and contractility of the heart during sepsis. [15, 16] Mediator production during polymicrobial sepsis is reduced in cardiomyocytes from C5aR- and C5L2-deficient mice. [16]

It has been shown that both C5a receptors, C5aR and C5L2, mediate the adverse functions of C5a when present in higher concentrations during sepsis. Mouse strains with targeted genetic deletion of C5aR or C5L2 are both protected during polymicrobial sepsis [17]. To date mouse strains with a double deletion phenotype for both receptors (C5aR-/- C5L2-/-) have not been studied since C5aR and C5L2 are expressed on the same chromosome, which would require de novo targeted deletion. Simultaneous blockade of C5aR plus C5L2 using antibodies against both receptors appears to be more protective that targeting either receptor alone. This suggests that C5aR and C5L2 act synergistically but may also have distinct biological profiles during sepsis. For example, signaling via C5L2 enhances the detrimental down-stream appearance of extracellular high mobility group protein B1 (HMGB1) and this effect is not shared by C5aR. [17]

In summary, our current knowledge obtained from experimental models of disease indicate that while low amounts of C5a may be required for clearance of pathogens during localized infection, an excessive generation of C5a may promote the progression to septic shock. If the current experimental findings obtained in small animal models, will correspond to the situation in human sepsis, cannot be fully answered at this time. Currently, a clinical trial is in progress which aims to investigate the effectiveness of neutralizing human C5a by a humanized antibody in sepsis. The outcomes of this trial will be helpful to assess the relevance of C5a as a potential target in human sepsis. Alternative strategies could involve blocking the C5a binding sites on the C5aR and/or C5L2 receptors by antibodies or the use of small molecule C5aR receptor antagonists.

Interleukin-27 (IL-27)

Non-covalent association of the protein chains p28 and Epstein Barr virus induced gene 3 (EBI3) forms a heterodimeric cytokine, IL-27. Structurally IL-27 belongs to the IL-12 family of cytokines. IL-27 is mainly produced by activated macrophages and dendritic cells when such cells encounter microbial products (LPS, viral nucleic acid). It is currently unclear if PMNs are also a relevant cellular source of IL-27 or rather are target cells, which bind IL-27 via the IL-27 receptor. In any case, the most abundant expression of the IL-27 receptor appears to be present on T cells. Ligation of IL-27 to the primary receptor chain (IL-27RA, WSX-1) initiates signaling via the gp130 receptor protein. Down-stream activation of STAT1 and STAT3 induces complex programs that alter expression of target genes. Most important, IL-27 can mediate the secretion of IL-10 by Th1 cells, Th2 cells, Th17 cells and T regulatory cells. Besides these anti-inflammatory properties, IL-27 can also induce IFNγ and support lymph node activation in germinal centers.

Construction of an Fc-IL-27RA receptor fusion protein was deployed for neutralization of IL-27 in polymicrobial sepsis following CLP in mice. Such Fc-IL-27RA treatment clearly improved mortality rates in C57BL/6 mice. {18] EBI3-deficient mice are also protected after CLP. Local bacterial growth in EBI3-deficient mice is better controlled because of a higher influx of leukocytes to the site of infection. Finally, IL-27RA-deficient mice display superior survival curves following endotoxic shock (Bosmann, unpublished findings).

Data from genome-wide transcriptional profiling has proposed IL-27 as novel diagnostic biomarker in sepsis. In critically ill children, the serum concentrations of IL-27 may discriminate between "sterile inflammation" and the presence of bacterial infections. [19] Although IL-27 as a biomarker was superior to procalcitonin in children, this was not observed in adults. [20] Nonetheless, dual testing of procalcitonin plus IL-27 may be a better predictor of sepsis in adults than either parameter alone.

The functional characteristics of IL-27 are quite unique in the way that IL-27 promotes inflammation in its acute phase, but silences chronic inflammation. One pathophysiologic dilemma of sepsis is thought to be acute hyperinflammation followed by chronic hypoinflammation/ immunosuppression. Hence, the kinetics of biological activities of IL-27 closely mimic the unfavorable picture of sepsis. In other words, therapeutic blockade of IL-27 may provide both protection from early tissue destructive inflammation and amelioration of the adverse long-lasting down-modulation of immunity (immunosuppression).

Neutrophil Extracellular Traps (NETs) and extracellular histones

It has been known for a long time that appearance of intracellular proteins in the extracellular compartments can disturb homeostasis, causing adverse biologic effects. For instance, massive trauma frequently causes rhabdomyolysis and hemolysis, which may progress to acute renal failure and disseminated intravascular coagulopathy. Since myosin and extracellular hemoglobin are highly cytotoxic, versatile mechanisms have evolved for rapid clearance of toxic hemoglobin from blood circulation.

By analogy, emerging evidence supports the concept that during sepsis nuclear proteins are released (actively and/or passively), resulting in detrimental effects. In 2004, the formation of neutrophil extracellular traps (NETs) during bacterial infections was first described. [21] NETs are structures of condensed chromatin (DNA/histones) and other antimicrobial proteins that are actively released from PMNs for the purpose of trapping and killing bacteria. NETs can also engulf fungal pathogens such as Candida albicans. Early on, the idea of NET formation faced considerable criticism within the scientific community, because artefacts of the employed in vitro imaging techniques could not be totally excluded. It was later demonstrated that NETs are also detectable in vivo using intra-vital microscopy. NETs not only are bactericidal but also have procoagulant activity. The intrinsic coagulation pathways are initiated by coagulation factor XII which is converted to factor XIIa on negatively charged surfaces of NETs. [22] Extracellular DNA/histones can be detected in histologic sections of blood clots and plasma from sub-human primates with deep vein thrombosis. [23] In addition, histones and DNA present in NETs can mediate platelet activation/aggregation, which can be prevented by the presence of DNase. [23] Alternatively, ligation of TLR4 on platelets can mediate PMN activation including NET formation during bacterial infection and sepsis. Plasma from patients with sepsis induces platelet-neutrophil interactions and triggers the appearance of NETs. [24] Thereby, NETs may provide a link between acute inflammation and the disturbances in coagulation observed in severe sepsis.

The formation of NETs is an active process and is different from the events underlying apoptosis or necrosis. In cell cultures of PMNs, NET formation can be induced by addition of bacteria, LPS, cytokines, chemokines such as IL-8 or PMA. [25] Several molecular processes involved in NET formation have been identified to date. For instance, production of ROS species is required for generation of NETs, since blockade of NADPH oxidase abrogates NET formation. [25] PMNs from patients with chronic granulomatous disease have greatly reduced NADPH oxidase activity and produce less NETs, unless ROS are substituted by addition of glucose oxidase. [25] Signaling via the Raf-MEK-ERK pathway precedes appearance of

NETs. [26] Down-stream of kinase signaling a complex mechanistic program is initiated which includes modification of chromatin structure. Arginine residues in core histone proteins are converted to citrulline by enzymes such as peptidylarginine deiminase 4 to facilitate chromatin decondensation (PAD4) [27]. PMNs derived from PAD4-deficient mice are incapable of forming NETs after incubation with chemokines or bacteria [28]. Accordingly, bacterial killing is defective in PAD4-deficient PMNs. On the other side, hypercitrullination decreases the bactericidal potency of histone proteins, suggesting that the citrullination is a prerequisite for the formation of NETs from nuclear chromatin rather than a requirement for the bactericidal capacity of NETs [28].

Extracellular histones are the major components of NETs but may also be released from dying non-immune cells in the course of sepsis or directly by blunt trauma before development of SIRS. When purified histone extracts are injected intravenously into healthy mice, rapid pathology ensues leading to death within minutes [29]. Extracellular histones are detectable in cell-free plasma of sub-human primates in the course of live E. coli sepsis [29]. Administration of neutralizing antibodies against histone H4 is protective in mouse models of endotoxic shock or polymicrobial sepsis after CLP [29]. In cell culture experiments, the incubation of endothelial cells with recombinant histone proteins leads to rapid Ca2+ influx and cell death. Interestingly, addition of activated protein C (APC) is protective in this experimental setting [29]. Inactivation of extracellular histones by APC-mediated cleavage may provide an explanation for the cytoprotective effects of APC in sepsis. Extracellular histones promote inflammation and production of cytokines after binding as endogenous ligands to TLR2 and TLR4 receptors [30].

Figure 2 gives a schematic overview of the pathophysiologic implications of endogenous cytotoxic factors in sepsis. Most likely, there is a broader role for extracellular histones and NETs as a common pathogenic mechanism in a wide spectrum of diseases beyond sepsis such as in acute lung injury/acute respiratory distress syndrome, thrombosis and autoimmune diseases.

High mobility group B 1 (HMGB1)

HMGB1 is an abundant protein in the cell nucleus, where it interacts with nucleosomes, histones and transcription factors for organizing chromatin structure and transcription. The highly conserved amino acid sequence of HMGB1 consists of 20% lysine residues as DNA-binding motifs. Upon hyperacetylation of its lysine residues HMGB1 translocates to the cytosol [31]. During inflammation monocytes and macrophages activated by pathogen-associated molecular patterns release HMGB1 to the extracellular spaces, where it acts in a cytokine-like fashion [32]. Other factors that induce HMGB1 release include proinflammatory cytokines (IL-1, TNFα) and apoptotic cell bodies. In detail, HMGB1 binds as an endogenous ligand ("danger signal") to the TLR4-receptor. The initiation of down-stream signaling cascades includes activation of NFκB and MAPK for regulation of target genes. HMGB1 induces its own gene expression and release with a delay of several hours. Important biological functions of HMGB1 are cytokine induction, activation of PMNs, chemotactic activity for myeloid cells, lymphocyte proliferation, disturbances in endothelial permeability and negative inotropic effects on cardiomyocytes.

In polymicrobial sepsis following CLP the serum concentration of HMGB1 slowly increase during a period of 24-48 h. This explains why neutralizing polyclonal or monoclonal antibodies against HMGB1 are protective even when given many hours after the onset of sepsis [33]. Likewise, blockade of HMGB1 is protective in models of SIRS when induced by massive trauma. Interception of HMGB1 during sepsis can also be accomplished by administration of recombinant HMGB1 A box, which acts as natural antagonist of cell binding of HMGB1. Several additional strategies to suppress HMGB1 release have been designed. Such efforts have included transcutaneous stimulation of the vagus nerve or injections with vasoactive intestinal peptide, ghrelin or urocortin.

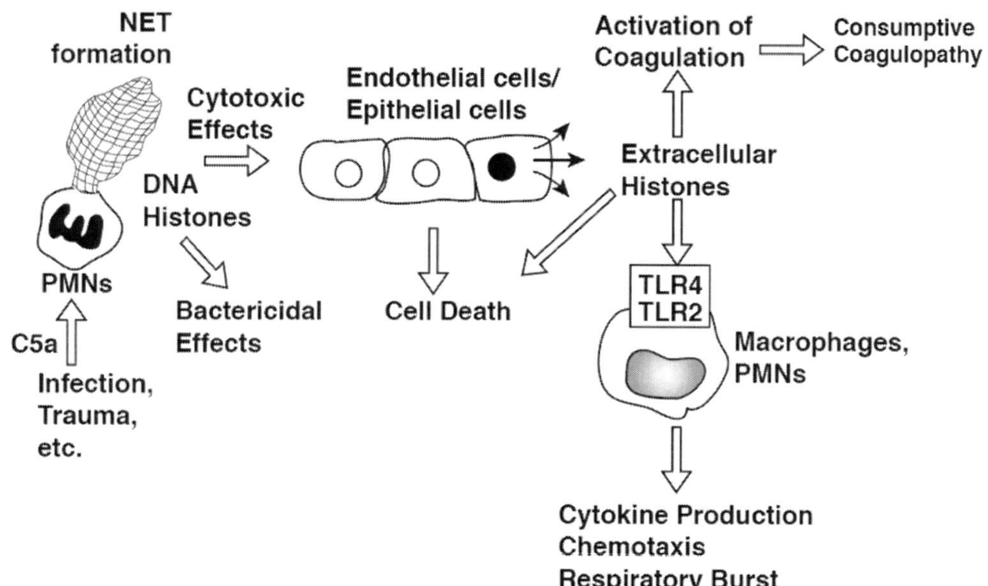

Figure 2. The concept of endogenous cytotoxic factors in sepsis. Infectious pathogens and non-infectious insults (e.g. hemorrhagic shock, polytrauma, etc.) trigger the release of neutrophil extracellular traps (NETs) from PMNs. NETs contain DNA and hypercitrullinated histones as predominant nuclear proteins. NETs trap and kill bacteria but are also cytotoxic to non-immune host cells. The loss of cellular integrity and cell death promotes the release of more histones into the extracellular spaces. Histones may also be released as a direct consequence of blunt trauma. Extracellular histones derived from NETs and non-immune cells activate the blood coagulation pathways and are endogenous ligands for innate pattern-recognition receptors. After binding to TLR4 and TLR2, histones induce cytokine production, chemotaxis and the respiratory burst. This results in progressive tissue destruction and organ dysfunction which may progress to multi-organ-failure and death.

Apoptosis of lymphocytes

At the later time points in the course of human sepsis a state of profound immunosuppression can occur. This is especially seen in individuals with advanced age and concomitant diseases. One hallmark of immunosuppression is a prolonged depletion of lymphocyte populations in spleen. The “cytokine storm”, bacterial and fungal factors of pathogenicity, hypoperfusion/catabolic metabolism and endogenous cytotoxic factors may all promote extensive apoptosis of lymphocyte populations.

T cell specific overexpression of the anti-apoptotic protein, Bcl-2, is protective against apoptosis of T cells during polymicrobial sepsis after CLP in mice and this results in better survival [34]. Likewise, siRNA knock-down of the death receptor Fas or caspase-8 improves survival in polymicrobial sepsis [35]. Apoptosis during polymicrobial sepsis can also be prevented by targeted thymic overexpression of IL-10 using adenoviral vectors [36]. On the other side, an anti-inflammatory cytokine profile (high IL-10/TNFα ratio) has been associated with a poor prognosis of infections in humans [37].

Apoptosis in septic patients occurs predominantly in lymphocytes and intestinal epithelial cells and is accompanied by increased presence of caspase-3 [38]. Lymphocyte apoptosis is noted in T cells (CD4, CD8) B cells (CD20) and NKT cells from septic patients via recruitment of caspase-8 and caspase-9 but this is not seen in non-septic control patients [39].

In a recent study, rapid post-mortem splenectomy was performed in 40 patients who died from severe sepsis with spleen from non-septic patients (brain death, trauma) serving as controls [40]. Immunosuppression in splenocytes from patients with sepsis was characterized by reduced numbers of CD4+ and CD8+ cells and a relative incapacity for cytokine production ex vivo.

Interleukin-7 (IL-7)

The cytokine IL-7 is a hematopoietic growth factor that is synthesized by non-lymphocytic cells such as stromal cells in the bone marrow, hepatocytes, epithelial cells, neurons and dendritic cells. IL-7 orchestrates the differentiation, proliferation and survival of T cells, B cells and NK cells (lymphoid cells). Hematopoietic stem cells are skewed by IL-7 for differentiation into lymphoid progenitor cells as opposed to differentiation into cells of the myeloid lineage. Thereby, IL-7 has the capacity to replenish the lymphocyte population following lymphocyte apoptosis in sepsis.

In polymicrobial sepsis of mice the administration of recombinant IL-7 effectively dampens lymphocyte apoptosis and improves survival rates [41]. IL-7 is also beneficial during fungal sepsis [42]. In another study leukocytes of sepsis patients were isolated and stimulated in vitro with IL-7. Such treatment with IL-7 restores the capacity of T cells for proliferation, activation of STAT5 and Bcl-2 signaling factors and production of Interferon-γ to levels comparable to leukocytes from healthy controls.

In clinical trials of cancer, administration of recombinant IL-7 resulted in 2-fold increases of spleen size and numbers of circulating CD4+ and CD8+ T cells, while numbers of T regulatory cells were diminished. Apparently, IL-7 is well tolerated, when given to patients with cancer or HIV-1. It will be interesting to see, if prospective clinical trials investigating IL-7 treatments in sepsis will show effectiveness without the development of side effects.

Programmed cell death protein 1 (PD-1)

PD-1 is a negative co-stimulatory membrane protein, which is expressed on activated T cells and B cells especially following persistent exposure to antigens. PD-1 can also be expressed on activated macrophages. The anti-inflammatory functions of PD-1 are activated by its ligand, PD-1L, which is also expressed on monocytes/macrophages. Activation of PD-1 is suppressive for a variety of T cell functions, including production of pro-inflammatory cytokines, T cell receptor-dependent cytotoxicity and T cell proliferation. Interception of the PD-1/PD-1L pathway can be accomplished by antagonistic anti-PD-1 antibodies or anti-PD-1L antibodies.

In mice with polymicrobial sepsis increasing expression patterns of PD-1 occur after 48 h [43]. More than 20% of CD4+ T cells and CD8+ T cells may be PD-1+ around one week after CLP. In this model blockade of PD-1 prevents sepsis-associated mortality even when administered 24 h after CLP [9]. Likewise, mice with genetic deficiency of PD-1 are protected from sepsis-induced lethality and display a lower burden of bacterial growth [44]. The beneficial effects of PD-1 are related to a reduced apoptosis of lymphocytes and innate immune cells. PD-1 blockade blocks the loss in mitochondrial BcL-xL, which is a member of the Bcl-2 family of anti-apoptotic proteins. Furthermore, PD-1 activation appears to be involved in the delayed-type hypersensitivity after sepsis, which is a surrogate marker for competent immune responses in sepsis survivors [43]. Anti-PD-L1 antibodies enhance bacterial clearance and result in higher concentrations of TNFα, IL-6 and lower IL-10 production [45].

In patients with sepsis the expression of PD-1 on peripheral blood T cells correlates with adverse outcomes such as more secondary nosocomial infections and deaths [46]. Abundant expression of PD-1 in sepsis results in decreased mitogen-induced proliferative capacities of T cells ex vivo. It remains to be seen, if blockade of PD-1/PD-1L would be protective in clinical trials of sepsis. At present anti-PD-1 treatments are already being investigated in clinical trials for the use in cancer patients, where PD-1 blockade appears to be well tolerated and induces clinical responses in 20-25% of cancer patients [47].

Current Challenges to Sepsis Research

The experimental approaches employed to uncover the molecular events of sepsis deserve closer attention. The current experimental models to study sepsis have several limitations. Novel clinical and experimental approaches may be needed to develop innovative strategies for the treatment of sepsis. There appears to be a disconnect between the currently used cell culture models and animal models in respect to their potential to adequately reflect the situation of sepsis in humans. In particular, these concerns have recently been raised by genome wide expression profiling of mouse models of sepsis when such data was compared with human sepsis [48].

In the past, bacterial endotoxins have been occasionally injected in low concentrations to healthy volunteers for investigating the acute systemic inflammatory response. These studies confirmed that lipopolysaccharides from bacteria directly induce the release of proinflammatory cytokines such as IL-1, IL-6 and TNFα in humans and cause clinical symptoms (tachycardia, fever) as found in sepsis. Naturally, the life-threatening nature of sepsis precludes the wide-spread use of experiments with human subjects because of ethical considerations. Experiments with non-human primates face comparable limitations but may not be avoidable to translate findings in small-animal models to human sepsis. Clinical observational and interventional sepsis trials are complicated by the heterogenicity of study populations and variations in sepsis definitions when used as inclusion criteria for controlled trials. Since sepsis is a common end point of a wide spectrum of clinical infections and conditions, the initial pathophysiologic events may vary substantially across individual cases. This may be especially applicable for patients with severe neutropenia, who regularly suffer from hematologic malignancies and often underwent aggressive chemotherapy shortly before the initial development of sepsis. In addition, the exact nature of the pathogenic microorganisms may be equally important as differences in the local site of primary infection (pulmonary versus abdominal) for the natural course of sepsis.

Experimental studies using small-animal models have been used for decades to define the molecular mechanisms in sepsis. Injections of endotoxins to rodents have been helpful to create a shock syndrome featuring many aspects of human sepsis. However, this approach is disadvantageous in respect to the absence of live pathogens and concomitant microbial factors of pathogenicity. For example, while pretreatments with anti-TNFα antibodies were highly protective in endotoxemia models of rodents, the use of anti-TNFα therapeutics in clinical trials of humans with sepsis overall failed to result in improved outcomes [49]. One factor in this equation may be the very early surge of TNFα during sepsis, which would require a rapid start of anti-TNF pharmaceuticals within the first few hours after diagnosis. Notably, the lethal doses of endotoxins are highly variable among different species. Mice and rats are much less sensitive to the toxic effects of lipopolysaccharides than humans or non-human primates.

Another discrepancy of human sepsis and small animal models in rodents is related to age. There is a strong correlation of the incidence of sepsis in humans with increasing age. On the other side, most experimental studies are being performed with juvenile healthy mice. Therefore, the overall health situation present in experimental animals often does not closely match with frail humans having multiple co-morbidities prior to the occurrence of infection and sepsis. In addition, most experimental studies on the immune responses during sepsis use models for gram-negative infections. Indeed, the currently available methodologies of acute gram-negative infections allow straight-forward investigations and are easily conducted. On the other side, experimental designs for gram-positive infections are often much more challenging. However, in humans gram-positive infections are predominant in frequency over gram-negative infections in sepsis. In future more experimental studies focusing on the pathologic mechanisms of gram-positive infections are necessary to adequately address the issues present in clinical settings.

In small animal models, wild type bacteria are typically used to induce infections. In human patients, bacteria encoding genes for multiple-antibiotic resistances are a common problem. Antibiotics are not always used in experimental models of sepsis (such as polymicrobial sepsis after CLP), and research animals often succumb during the early proinflammatory state of sepsis. In contrast, human patients often survive the acute proinflammatory phase of sepsis. This is due to substantial advances in critical care medicine including treatment regimens of antibiotics, vasopressors, hemodialysis/hemofiltration and mechanical ventilation the latter requiring the concomitant use of sedatives. After initial stabilization human sepsis patients often develop a state of prolonged immunosuppression, which leaves them susceptible for opportunistic infections and death at later time points.

In summary, one future challenge of sepsis research will be to close the gap between experimental findings and the pathogenesis and progression of human sepsis under advanced treatment modalities. New experimental models that more closely match with the situation in human patients would be tremendously helpful. For example, "humanized mice" could be generated by transplantation of human immune cells in immune compromised mice (e.g. SCID, NSG) and this may allow better simulation of human sepsis in small animal models. A thoughtful choice of clinically relevant pathogens (bacterial, fungal) will be equally important as the selection of appropriate administration routes for these pathogens.

Finally, there may be no "magic bullet" to uniformly cure all categories of human sepsis. More likely the different forms of sepsis such as gram-negative sepsis, gram-positive sepsis, fungal sepsis, neutropenic sepsis, pneumonia-induced sepsis, sepsis of the elderly, trauma-induced sepsis, burn-induced sepsis and SIRS may each require individual treatment strategies focusing on different molecular targets.

Concluding Remarks

In the past two decades considerable advance have been made in understanding the molecular mechanisms of sepsis. The future challenges will be to validate these findings in the setting of clinical sepsis in humans. In addition, advanced methodologies such as genome wide sequencing approaches and intra-vital imaging technologies may open new avenues for sepsis research in the future. Considerable progress has been made in critical care medical treatment of sepsis. New mechanical devices including a more wide-spread use of high-frequency lung ventilation and extracorporal membrane oxygenation may be helpful for sub-groups of patients with severe sepsis.

The hopes for an immediate availability of specific pharmaceuticals for the treatment of sepsis have been nullified by the withdrawal of recombinant activated protein C from the drug market a few years ago.

The major issues of many pharmaceuticals designed against sepsis are high costs and lack of effectiveness rather than toxicity or low safety profiles. A great deal of frustration has swept over the landscape of pharmaceutical industries regarding the willingness to invest large amounts of finance in the sepsis field. Likewise, academic research in the sepsis field is underfinanced with only a low proportion of governmental research budgets dedicated to investigate this vicious disease. Giving the high burden of sepsis on public health this is more than surprising. A potential explanation for this phenomenon may be the low public awareness about sepsis.

Unlike patients with chronic diseases such as cancer or HIV, who are living as members of society for years, critically ill sepsis patient are segregated on intensive care units, where they may die within a few days or weeks. Moreover, it appears that in the public perception of non-medical individuals it is widely believed that bacterial infections should be easily curable by antibiotics. Therefore, the existence of high numbers of nosocomial infections and their complications appear not to be a "good advertisement" for certain hospitals and health systems.

Hence, there may be a subtle notion of not making too much mention of sepsis in public discussions. This needs to be changed. Campaigns to raise the general awareness about sepsis may be helpful for starting public debates for allocating more resources to research, treatment and prevention of sepsis in industrialized countries.

Acknowledgments

P.A.W. was supported by grants from the U.S. National Institutes of Health (GM-29507, GM-61656). M.B. was supported by grants of the Federal Ministry of Education and Research (01EO1003), the Deutsche Forschungsgemeinschaft (BO 3482/3-1), the MAIFOR Program of the University Medical Center Mainz, the B. Braun Foundation and by a Marie Curie Career Integration Grant of the European Union (334486). We thank Sue Scott, Beverly Schumann and Robin Kunkel for assistance in the preparation of the manuscript.

References

[1] Adhikari, N. K., Fowler, R. A., Bhagwanjee, S. & Rubenfeld, G. D. (2010). Critical care and the global burden of critical illness in adults. *Lancet*, *376*, 1339-1346.

[2] Martin, G. S., Mannino, D. M., Eaton, S. & Moss, M. (2003). The epidemiology of sepsis in the United States from 1979 through 2000. *New England Journal of Medicine*, *348*, 1546-1554.

[3] Wong, C. H., Jenne, C. N., Petri, B., Chrobok, N. L. & Kubes, P. (2013). Nucleation of platelets with blood-borne pathogens on Kupffer cells precedes other innate immunity and contributes to bacterial clearance. *Nat Immunol*, *14*, 785-792.

[4] Andersson, U. & Tracey, K. J. (2012). Neural reflexes in inflammation and immunity. *J Exp Med*, *209*, 1057-1068.

[5] Tracey, K. J. (2009). Reflex control of immunity. *Nat Rev Immunol*, *9*, 418-428.

[6] Rosas-Ballina, M., Olofsson, P. S., Ochani, M., Valdes-Ferrer, S. I., Levine, Y. A., Reardon, C., Tusche, M. W., Pavlov, V. A., Andersson, U., Chavan, S., Mak, T. W. & Tracey, K. J. (2011). Acetylcholine-synthesizing T cells relay neural signals in a vagus nerve circuit. *Science*, *334*, 98-101.

[7] Matteoli, G., Gomez-Pinilla, P. J., Nemethova, A., Di Giovangiulio, M., Cailotto, C., van Bree, S. H., Michel, K., Tracey, K. J., Schemann, M., Boesmans, W., Vanden Berghe, P. & Boeckxstaens, G. E. (2013). A distinct vagal anti-inflammatory pathway modulates intestinal muscularis resident macrophages independent of the spleen. *Gut*.

[8] Kessler, W., Diedrich, S., Menges, P., Ebker, T., Nielson, M., Partecke, L. I., Traeger, T., Cziupka, K., van der Linde, J., Puls, R., Busemann, A., Heidecke, C. D. & Maier, S. (2012). The role of the vagus nerve: modulation of the inflammatory reaction in murine polymicrobial sepsis. *Mediators of inflammation*, 2012, 467620.

[9] van Westerloo, D. J., Giebelen, I. A., Florquin, S., Daalhuisen, J., Bruno, M. J., de Vos, A. F., Tracey, K. J. & van der Poll, T. (2005). The cholinergic anti-inflammatory pathway regulates the host response during septic peritonitis. *J Infect Dis*, *191*, 2138-2148.

[10] Ricklin, D., Hajishengallis, G., Yang, K. & Lambris, J. D. (2010). Complement: a key system for immune surveillance and homeostasis. *Nat Immunol*, *11*, 785-797.

[11] Bosmann, M. & Ward, P. A. (2012). Role of C3, C5 and anaphylatoxin receptors in acute lung injury and in sepsis. *Advances in experimental medicine and biology*, *946*, 147-159.

[12] Czermak, B. J., Sarma, V., Pierson, C. L., Warner, R. L., Huber-Lang, M., Bless, N. M., Schmal, H., Friedl, H. P. & Ward, P. A. (1999). Protective effects of C5a blockade in sepsis. *Nature Medicine*, *5*, 788-792.

[13] Bosmann, M., Sarma, J. V., Atefi, G., Zetoune, F. S. & Ward, P. A. (2012). Evidence for anti-inflammatory effects of C5a on the innate IL-17A/IL-23 axis. *FASEB J*, *26*, 1640-1651.

[14] Laudes, I. J., Chu, J. C., Sikranth, S., Huber-Lang, M., Guo, R. F., Riedemann, N., Sarma, J. V., Schmaier, A. H. & Ward, P. A. (2002). Anti-c5a ameliorates coagulation/fibrinolytic protein changes in a rat model of sepsis. *Am J Pathol*, *160*, 1867-1875.

[15] Niederbichler, A. D., Hoesel, L. M., Westfall, M. V., Gao, H. W., Ipaktchi, K. R., Sun, L., Zetoune, F. S., Su, G. L., Arbabi, S., Sarma, J. V., Wang, S. C., Hemmila, M. R. & Ward, P. A. (2006). An essential role for complement C5a in the pathogenesis of septic cardiac dysfunction. *Journal of Experimental Medicine*, *203*, 53-61.

[16] Atefi, G., Zetoune, F. S., Herron, T. J., Jalife, J., Bosmann, M., Al-Aref, R., Sarma, J. V. & Ward, P. A. (2011). Complement dependency of cardiomyocyte release of mediators during sepsis. *The FASEB journal : official publication of the Federation of American Societies for Experimental Biology.*

[17] Rittirsch, D., Flierl, M. A., Nadeau, B. A., Day, D. E., Huber-Lang, M., Mackay, C. R., Zetoune, F. S., Gerard, N. P., Cianflone, K., Kohl, J., Gerard, C., Sarma, J. V. & Ward, P. A. (2008). Functional roles for C5a receptors in sepsis. *Nature Medicine*, *14*, 551-557.

[18] Wirtz, S., Tubbe, I., Galle, P. R., Schild, H. J., Birkenbach, M., Blumberg, R. S. & Neurath, M. F. (2006). Protection from lethal septic peritonitis by neutralizing the biological function of interleukin 27. *Journal of Experimental Medicine*, *203*, 1875-1881.

[19] Wong, H. R., Cvijanovich, N. Z., Hall, M., Allen, G. L., Thomas, N. J., Freishtat, R. J., Anas, N., Meyer, K., Checchia, P. A., Lin, R., Bigham, M. T., Sen, A., Nowak, J., Quasney, M., Henricksen, J. W., Chopra, A., Banschbach, S., Beckman, E., Harmon, K., Lahni, P. & Shanley, T. P. (2012). Interleukin-27 is a novel candidate diagnostic biomarker for bacterial infection in critically ill children. *Critical care*, *16*, R213.

[20] Wong, H. R., Lindsell, C. J., Lahni, P., Hart, K. W. & Gibot, S. (2013). Interleukin-27 as a sepsis diagnostic biomarker in critically ill adults. *Shock*.

[21] Brinkmann, V., Reichard, U., Goosmann, C., Fauler, B., Uhlemann, Y., Weiss, D. S., Weinrauch, Y. & Zychlinsky, A. (2004). Neutrophil extracellular traps kill bacteria. *Science*, *303*, 1532-1535.

[22] von Bruhl, M. L., Stark, K., Steinhart, A., Chandraratne, S., Konrad, I., Lorenz, M., Khandoga, A., Tirniceriu, A., Coletti, R., Kollnberger, M., Byrne, R. A., Laitinen, I., Walch, A., Brill, A., Pfeiler, S., Manukyan, D., Braun, S., Lange, P., Riegger, J., Ware, J., Eckart, A., Haidari, S., Rudelius, M., Schulz, C., Echtler, K., Brinkmann, V., Schwaiger, M., Preissner, K. T., Wagner, D. D., Mackman, N., Engelmann, B. & Massberg, S. (2012). Monocytes, neutrophils, and platelets cooperate to initiate and propagate venous thrombosis in mice in vivo. *J Exp Med*, *209*, 819-835.

[23] Fuchs, T. A., Brill, A., Duerschmied, D., Schatzberg, D., Monestier, M., Myers, D. D., Jr., Wrobleski, S. K., Wakefield, T. W., Hartwig, J. H. & Wagner, D. D. (2010). Extracellular DNA traps promote thrombosis. *Proc Natl Acad Sci U S A*, *107*, 15880-15885.

[24] Clark, S. R., Ma, A. C., Tavener, S. A., McDonald, B., Goodarzi, Z., Kelly, M. M., Patel, K. D., Chakrabarti, S., McAvoy, E., Sinclair, G. D., Keys, E. M., Allen-Vercoe, E., Devinney, R., Doig, C. J., Green, F. H. & Kubes, P. (2007). Platelet TLR4 activates neutrophil extracellular traps to ensnare bacteria in septic blood. *Nat Med*, *13*, 463-469.

[25] Fuchs, T. A., Abed, U., Goosmann, C., Hurwitz, R., Schulze, I., Wahn, V., Weinrauch, Y., Brinkmann, V. & Zychlinsky, A. (2007). Novel cell death program leads to neutrophil extracellular traps. *The Journal of cell biology*, *176*, 231-241.

[26] Hakkim, A., Fuchs, T. A., Martinez, N. E., Hess, S., Prinz, H., Zychlinsky, A. & Waldmann, H. (2011). Activation of the Raf-MEK-ERK pathway is required for neutrophil extracellular trap formation. *Nature chemical biology*, *7*, 75-77.

[27] Neeli, I., Khan, S. N. & Radic, M. (2008). Histone deimination as a response to inflammatory stimuli in neutrophils. *J Immunol*, *180*, 1895-1902.

[28] Li, P., Li, M., Lindberg, M. R., Kennett, M. J., Xiong, N. & Wang, Y. (2010). PAD4 is essential for antibacterial innate immunity mediated by neutrophil extracellular traps. *J Exp Med*, *207*, 1853-1862.

[29] Xu, J., Zhang, X., Pelayo, R., Monestier, M., Ammollo, C. T., Semeraro, F., Taylor, F. B., Esmon, N. L., Lupu, F. & Esmon, C. T. (2009). Extracellular histones are major mediators of death in sepsis. *Nat Med*, *15*, 1318-1321.

[30] Xu, J., Zhang, X., Monestier, M., Esmon, N. L. & Esmon, C. T. (2011). Extracellular histones are mediators of death through TLR2 and TLR4 in mouse fatal liver injury. *J Immunol*, *187*, 2626-2631.

[31] Klune, J. R., Dhupar, R., Cardinal, J., Billiar, T. R. & Tsung, A. (2008). HMGB1: endogenous danger signaling. *Molecular medicine*, *14*, 476-484.

[32] Andersson, U. & Tracey, K. J. (2011). HMGB1 is a therapeutic target for sterile inflammation and infection. *Annu Rev Immunol*, *29*, 139-162.

[33] Qin, S., Wang, H., Yuan, R., Li, H., Ochani, M., Ochani, K., Rosas-Ballina, M., Czura, C. J., Huston, J. M., Miller, E., Lin, X., Sherry, B., Kumar, A., Larosa, G., Newman, W., Tracey, K. J. & Yang, H. (2006). Role of HMGB1 in apoptosis-mediated sepsis lethality. *J Exp Med*, *203*, 1637-1642.

[34] Hotchkiss, R. S., Swanson, P. E., Knudson, C. M., Chang, K. C., Cobb, J. P., Osborne, D. F., Zollner, K. M., Buchman, T. G., Korsmeyer, S. J. & Karl, I. E. (1999). Overexpression of Bcl-2 in transgenic mice decreases apoptosis and improves survival in sepsis. *J Immunol*, *162*, 4148-4156.

[35] Wesche-Soldato, D. E., Chung, C. S., Lomas-Neira, J., Doughty, L. A., Gregory, S. H. & Ayala, A. (2005). In vivo delivery of caspase-8 or Fas siRNA improves the survival of septic mice. *Blood*, *106*, 2295-2301.

[36] Oberholzer, C., Oberholzer, A., Bahjat, F. R., Minter, R. M., Tannahill, C. L., Abouhamze, A., LaFace, D., Hutchins, B., Clare-Salzler, M. J. & Moldawer, L. L. (2001). Targeted adenovirus-induced expression of IL-10 decreases thymic apoptosis and improves survival in murine sepsis. *Proc Natl Acad Sci U S A*, *98*, 11503-11508

[37] van Dissel, J. T., van Langevelde, P., Westendorp, R. G., Kwappenberg, K. & Frolich, M. (1998). Anti-inflammatory cytokine profile and mortality in febrile patients. *Lancet*, *351*, 950-953.

[38] Hotchkiss, R. S., Swanson, P. E., Freeman, B. D., Tinsley, K. W., Cobb, J. P., Matuschak, G. M., Buchman, T. G. & Karl, I. E. (1999). Apoptotic cell death in patients with sepsis, shock, and multiple organ dysfunction. *Crit Care Med*, *27*, 1230-1251.

[39] Hotchkiss, R. S., Osmon, S. B., Chang, K. C., Wagner, T. H., Coopersmith, C. M. & Karl, I. E. (2005). Accelerated lymphocyte death in sepsis occurs by both the death receptor and mitochondrial pathways. *J Immunol*, *174*, 5110-5118.

[40] Boomer, J. S., To, K., Chang, K. C., Takasu, O., Osborne, D. F., Walton, A. H., Bricker, T. L., Jarman, S. D., 2nd, Kreisel, D., Krupnick, A. S., Srivastava, A., Swanson, P. E., Green, J. M. & Hotchkiss, R. S. (2011). Immunosuppression in patients

who die of sepsis and multiple organ failure. *JAMA : the journal of the American Medical Association, 306*, 2594-2605.

[41] Unsinger, J., McGlynn, M., Kasten, K. R., Hoekzema, A. S., Watanabe, E., Muenzer, J. T., McDonough, J. S., Tschoep, J., Ferguson, T. A., McDunn, J. E., Morre, M., Hildeman, D. A., Caldwell, C. C. & Hotchkiss, R. S. (2010). IL-7 promotes T cell viability, trafficking, and functionality and improves survival in sepsis. *J Immunol, 184*, 3768-3779.

[42] Unsinger, J., Burnham, C. A., McDonough, J., Morre, M., Prakash, P. S., Caldwell, C. C., Dunne, W. M., Jr. & Hotchkiss, R. S. (2012). Interleukin-7 ameliorates immune dysfunction and improves survival in a 2-hit model of fungal sepsis. *J Infect Dis, 206*, 606-616.

[43] Brahmamdam, P., Inoue, S., Unsinger, J., Chang, K. C., McDunn, J. E. & Hotchkiss, R. S. (2010). Delayed administration of anti-PD-1 antibody reverses immune dysfunction and improves survival during sepsis. *J Leukoc Biol, 88*, 233-240.

[44] Huang, X., Venet, F., Wang, Y. L., Lepape, A., Yuan, Z., Chen, Y., Swan, R., Kherouf, H., Monneret, G., Chung, C. S. & Ayala, A. (2009). PD-1 expression by macrophages plays a pathologic role in altering microbial clearance and the innate inflammatory response to sepsis. *Proc Natl Acad Sci U S A, 106*, 6303-6308.

[45] Zhang, Y., Zhou, Y., Lou, J., Li, J., Bo, L., Zhu, K., Wan, X., Deng, X. & Cai, Z. (2010). PD-L1 blockade improves survival in experimental sepsis by inhibiting lymphocyte apoptosis and reversing monocyte dysfunction. *Critical care, 14*, R220.

[46] Guignant, C., Lepape, A., Huang, X., Kherouf, H., Denis, L., Poitevin, F., Malcus, C., Cheron, A., Allaouchiche, B., Gueyffier, F., Ayala, A., Monneret, G. & Venet, F. (2011). Programmed death-1 levels correlate with increased mortality, nosocomial infection and immune dysfunctions in septic shock patients. *Critical care, 15*, R99.

[47] Topalian, S. L., Hodi, F. S., Brahmer, J. R., Gettinger, S. N., Smith, D. C., McDermott, D. F., Powderly, J. D., Carvajal, R. D., Sosman, J. A., Atkins, M. B., Leming, P. D., Spigel, D. R., Antonia, S. J., Horn, L., Drake, C. G., Pardoll, D. M., Chen, L., Sharfman, W. H., Anders, R. A., Taube, J. M., McMiller, T. L., Xu, H., Korman, A. J., Jure-Kunkel, M., Agrawal, S., McDonald, D., Kollia, G. D., Gupta, A., Wigginton, J. M. & Sznol, M. (2012). Safety, activity, and immune correlates of anti-PD-1 antibody in cancer. *N Engl J Med, 366*, 2443-2454.

[48] Seok, J., Warren, H. S., Cuenca, A. G., Mindrinos, M. N., Baker, H. V., Xu, W., Richards, D. R., McDonald-Smith, G. P., Gao, H., Hennessy, L., Finnerty, C. C., Lopez, C. M., Honari, S., Moore, E. E., Minei, J. P., Cuschieri, J., Bankey, P. E., Johnson, J. L., Sperry, J., Nathens, A. B., Billiar, T. R., West, M. A., Jeschke, M. G., Klein, M. B., Gamelli, R. L., Gibran, N. S., Brownstein, B. H., Miller-Graziano, C., Calvano, S. E., Mason, P. H., Cobb, J. P., Rahme, L. G., Lowry, S. F., Maier, R. V., Moldawer, L. L., Herndon, D. N., Davis, R. W., Xiao, W., Tompkins, R. G., Inflammation & Host Response to Injury, L. S. C. R. P. (2013). Genomic responses in mouse models poorly mimic human inflammatory diseases. *Proc Natl Acad Sci U S A, 110*, 3507-3512.

[49] Reinhart, K. & Karzai, W. (2001). Anti-tumor necrosis factor therapy in sepsis: update on clinical trials and lessons learned. *Crit Care Med, 29*, S121-125.

[50] Marti-Carvajal, A. J., Sola, I., Gluud, C., Lathyris, D. & Cardona, A. F. (2012). Human recombinant protein C for severe sepsis and septic shock in adult and paediatric patients. *The Cochrane database of systematic reviews*, *12*, CD004388.

[51] Cohen, J. (1999). Adjunctive therapy in sepsis: a critical analysis of the clinical trial programme. *British medical bulletin*, *55*, 212-225.

[52] Fisher, C. J., Jr., Dhainaut, J. F., Opal, S. M., Pribble, J. P., Balk, R. A., Slotman, G. J., Iberti, T. J., Rackow, E. C., Shapiro, M. J., Greenman, R. L. et al., (1994). Recombinant human interleukin 1 receptor antagonist in the treatment of patients with sepsis syndrome. Results from a randomized, double-blind, placebo-controlled trial. Phase III rhIL-1ra Sepsis Syndrome Study Group. *JAMA : the journal of the American Medical Association*, *271*, 1836-1843.

[53] Opal, S. M., Fisher, C. J., Jr., Dhainaut, J. F., Vincent, J. L., Brase, R., Lowry, S. F., Sadoff, J. C., Slotman, G. J., Levy, H., Balk, R. A., Shelly, M. P., Pribble, J. P., LaBrecque, J. F., Lookabaugh, J., Donovan, H., Dubin, H., Baughman, R., Norman, J., DeMaria, E., Matzel, K., Abraham, E. & Seneff, M. (1997). Confirmatory interleukin-1 receptor antagonist trial in severe sepsis: a phase III, randomized, double-blind, placebo-controlled, multicenter trial. The Interleukin-1 Receptor Antagonist Sepsis Investigator Group. *Crit Care Med*, *25*, 1115-1124.

[54] Bernard, G. R., Wheeler, A. P., Russell, J. A., Schein, R., Summer, W. R., Steinberg, K. P., Fulkerson, W. J., Wright, P. E., Christman, B. W., Dupont, W. D., Higgins, S. B. & Swindell, B. B. (1997). The effects of ibuprofen on the physiology and survival of patients with sepsis. The Ibuprofen in Sepsis Study Group. *N Engl J Med*, *336*, 912-918.

[55] Memis, D., Karamanlioglu, B., Turan, A., Koyuncu, O. & Pamukcu, Z. (2004). Effects of lornoxicam on the physiology of severe sepsis. *Critical care*, *8*, R474-482.

[56] Avontuur, J. A., Tutein Nolthenius, R. P., van Bodegom, J. W. & Bruining, H. A. (1998). Prolonged inhibition of nitric oxide synthesis in severe septic shock: a clinical study. *Crit Care Med*, *26*, 660-667.

[57] Spies, C. D., Reinhart, K., Witt, I., Meier-Hellmann, A., Hannemann, L., Bredle, D. L. & Schaffartzik, W. (1994). Influence of N-acetylcysteine on indirect indicators of tissue oxygenation in septic shock patients: results from a prospective, randomized, double-blind study. *Crit Care Med*, *22*, 1738-1746.

In: Sepsis
Editor: Nancy Khardori
ISBN: 978-1-63117-244-1

Chapter 2

Myocardial Dysfunction in Sepsis: Role of Apelin, a Novel Promising Molecule

Robert Dumaine, Ph.D., Michaël Biet, Ph.D., David Coquerel, MsC, and Olivier Lesur[1] , M.D., Ph.D. [*]
[1]Dept de Médecine (Soins Intensifs Médicaux) and Dept de Physiologie-Biophysique, Université de Sherbrooke, Québec, Canada

Abstract

Severe sepsis and septic shock are prevalent worldwide and the heart is one of the most threatened organs in a multiple organ failure profile. Dobutamine is the recommended β-adrenergic inotropic drug to support sepsis-induced myocardial dysfunction after fluid resuscitation when failure is obvious. However, alternative supportive and safer therapies are sought. For instance, combined milrinone and metoprolol therapy may be an effective alternative therapy but Apelin is another promising molecule. Apelin is a natural endogenous neuropeptide, centrally and peripherally counter regulated by arginine-vasopressin. Indeed, through its highly expressed specific receptor APJ-R, Apelin can improve heart contractility and relaxation in both normal and failing hearts, and is a vasodilator potentially reducing after-load and facilitating ventricular work.

Introduction

Almost nothing is known as to Apelin involvement in sepsis and its potential impact on outcome and sepsis – induced myocardial dysfunction. In this short review, we will describe:

[*] Correspondence: Olivier Lesur MD, PhD; 3001, 12th Avenue Nord; Sherbrooke, Québec Canada; J1H 5N4; Olivier.Lesur@USherbrooke.ca.

1) Sepsis-induced myocardial dysfunction, 2) the new history of Apelin, 3) Apelin as a critical regulator of vascular tone in a Nitric Oxide (NO)-dependent manner, 4) Apelin-related improvement of cardiac contractility, 5) Apelin as a cardioprotector in heart disease, 6) Apelin as a modulator of heart electrical activity, 7) Apelin commitment in cardiac development and angiogenesis, 8) Apelin as a participant in fluid homeostasis, 9) other physiological actions of Apelin, 10) potential impacts of Apelin in sepsis-induced myocardial dysfunctions.

1. Sepsis-Induced Myocardial Dysfunction

Severe sepsis strikes an estimated 750,000 people in USA each year and this rate is expected to rise to 1 million cases a year and was recently estimated to double (2006-2009) as the population ages. [1] Septic shock (i.e., the archetypal catastrophic form of severe sepsis) is a leading cause of death for patients admitted in ICUs. [1] A similar number of deaths per year to that reported from acute myocardial infarction, lung or breast cancers have been recently observed for severe sepsis or septic shock in the USA. [2-3] Septic shock is defined by the association of documented infection with decreased arterial blood pressure below 60mm Hg in spite of 1L solute infusion and need of vasopressors. [2,4] Morbidity and mortality rates of septic shock are rather high (20-90%) and Multiple Organ Failure occurs rapidly with the increasing severity of the septic condition [2,4]. In this context, one of the most limiting organ often remains the heart (or the cardiovascular status), demonstrating refractory pump failure with major systolic and/or diastolic dysfunction(s). [2,4] It is associated with a significant increased mortality rate of 70 to 90% in comparison with the 20-30% mortality in septic patients without cardiovascular impairment. [5] Recently, up to ⅔ and ¼ of patients in septic shock, exhibited global left ventricular hyperkinesia'-relaxation impairments in the first 48hrs of sepsis onset [6,7-8], and a left ventricular dilation is usually observed as a compensatory mechanism to maintain cardiac output which has also been noted in endotoxin [lipopolysaccharides: LPS]-challenged volunteers-. [9-10]

In the "surviving sepsis campaign" guidelines [11], dobutamine is the actual recommended β-adrenergic inotropic drug to support sepsis-induced myocardial dysfunction after fluid resuscitation when cardiac output index is still low because dobutamine's cardiovascular response predicts outcome in septic shock. [12] Alternative supportive and safer therapies are however mandatory because: 1) only 35-45% of septic patients do respond to dobutamine, and 2) numerous side-effects of dobutamine can be observed, including potential harmful impact on cardiomyocyte function. [12-13] Combined milrinone and metoprolol therapy may be an effective alternative therapy but still lacks data evidence.

Direct cardiomyocyte insult is not the exclusive hallmark of "macro" ischemia /reperfusion, and severe sepsis or septic shock is injury providers for heart walls with enhanced membrane permeability/ injury. [14-16] Indeed, rising blood cardiac troponin I (cTnI) as an early sensitive marker of acute coronary syndromes, has also been documented in stretch-super imposed hemodynamic conditions to ventricular walls and in sepsis. [7-8, 17-19] Correlations have been even reported between cTnI levels and cardiac dysfunction in septic shock. [18-19] In addition, Tavernier et al [20], demonstrated experimentally a significant increased myocardial expression of activated phosphorylated cTnI several hours after LPS challenge, which is a fine-tune marker of reduced cardiac myofilament Ca^{2+} response and a signal of disturbed cardiac muscle shortening and relaxation kinetics.

Infiltration of myocardial tissues by both polymorphonuclear neutrophil (PMN) recruitment/spillover and activated monocyte-macrophages, together with cellular and interstitial edema, are critical components of heart dysfunction in human and experimental sepsis. [21-29] Locally and systemically-produced cytokines such as MIF, or TNF-α, amplify this inflammatory cascade, leading to vital organ dysfunction including heart. [30-31] Neutralizing specifically these cytokines may be useful. For instance, blocking MIF almost restores cardiac function after LPS challenge or burn injury with extended tissue damage, and can improve autoimmune myocarditis and ischemic heart [22, 30, 32], leading to improved survival. [33] Endogenous anti-inflammatory molecules which are produced by or target heart may also help in controlling myocardial burst. Acute myocardial edema affects both systolic and diastolic functions, with underestimated impact on heart compliance and relaxation. [34-35] With sophistication of echographic and MRI devices, this component of structural myocardial wall alterations is now measurable. [35-36] Edema can occur at the interstitial/intercellular level and/or at the cellular level (cell swelling), and a first line protection for the heart is the endothelial glycocalyx. [37-38] LPS challenge and hypovolemic shock induce interstitial/intercellular space enlargement in rat hearts with altered endothelial resistance. [39-41] Indeed the heart is the fourth leaking vital organ (with kidney, liver and lung) several hours after LPS challenge; bacteriemia or cecal ligation puncture. [28,40], and disturbance in water and solutes handling are likely to be involved in myocardial dysfunction. In this respect, aquaporin-1 is the most expressed aquaporin in human intramural myocardial capillaries and sarcolemma membranes [42-43], and displays location within transverse tubules which are invaginations of the surface membrane of cardiomyocytes and intercalated discs that originate at the Z-lines/bands. Both play an essential role in the excitation-contraction coupling and communication with the extracellular space. Anemia and ischemia-reperfusion enhance aquaporin-1myocardial expression [44-45], and hyperosmotic stimuli induce aquaporin-1recruitment to plasma membrane. [46] Chloride channels and more specifically, swelling-activated chloride currents ($I_{CL\text{-swell}}$ currents) are also committed in cell volume regulation and apoptosis. [47-48] Sustained myocardial dysfunction in LPS-challenged hearts is associated with shortened action potential duration. [49] This can be initially protective –such as in acute ischemia- but leads to sodium and chloride accumulation with intracellular water content increase. In this respect, $I_{CL\text{-swell}}$ currents are activated in cardiomyocytes from endotoxic shock [50], and are potentially involved in wall edema-induced myocardial dysfunction. [51]

Apoptosis is a physiological and specific cell death process often dysregulated in inflammation and injury. [52] Enhanced apoptosis leads to delayed repair processes and to major life-threatening organ dysfunction. Cardiomyocyte apoptosis has gained increasing interest for several years in the understanding of ischemic disease and other cardiomyopathies. [53-55,31] In endotoxic models, MIF as well as TNF-α are apoptotic for cardiomyocytes [56-57], cardiac apoptosis and myocardial function are tightly related; and neutralization of MIF or TNF-α reverses apoptotic streams and restores cardiac function. [58,31] In most cases, the initiation and execution phases of the apoptotic processes involve activation of a family of proteases called caspases. The executioner caspase 3 is critical in the degradation phase. Indeed, both caspase 3 activity and downstream DNA fragmentation profile are generally well correlated and increased early in LPS-challenged heart [53-63], and are useful general markers of the apoptotic level. Two main apoptotic pathways converge on the activation of effector caspases. [64] The first one integrates different pro-apoptotic signals at the mitochondrial level (with release of cytochrome *c*) and the second one is independent of mitochondria and involves activation of procaspases by death receptors. [64] Other pathways exist that can counterbalance the above and prevent cellular death processes.

In parallel, no commitment in function and myocardial cell survival is well known. Increased expression of cardiac iNOS is observed in most endotoxic models with myocardial dysfunction, as well as in human septic hearts, and is a catalyzer of apoptosis. [60] NOS inhibition however failed to reverse septic shock in a phase III clinical trial using L-NMMA. The nonselectivity of L-NMMA treatment-induced unbalance, especially as to iNOS and constitutive eNOS/neuronal nitric oxide synthase (nNOS) expression, has been suggested to explain this flaw. In this respect, eNOS is hugely expressed in the heart and is the one which constitutively shares inotropic & lusitropic activities, on the opposite of iNOS. [65] From this standpoint, sera from patients with severe heart failure down-regulate eNOS with pro-apoptotic impact on endothelial cells [66], erythropoietin drives eNOS-mediated cardioprotection. [67] Data on nNOS in the cardiac system are more puzzling. Overall, at the heart level nNOS is an autocrine regulator of myocardial inotropy/relaxation [68-70] and is contributive to locally inhibit inflammation induced by LPS, improving cardiac function. [71] Xu et al located cardiac muscle nNOS in the sarcoplasmic reticulum (SR) where it is committed in Ca^{2+} active transport [72], a way by-which many inotropic molecules work . Much less is known as to nNOS impact on apoptosis, but a double-edged sword effect of the tandem nNOS/iNOS expression has been suggested.

2. The New History of Apelin

Apelin is an endogenous bioactive peptide which is expressed in a wide variety of tissues and binds to the angiotensin-like 1 (APJ) receptor. [73-74] In 1993, O'Dowd *et al* discovered a 700 base pair gene coding for a protein-receptor of 380 aminoacids (AA) with high similarities to the angiotensin II type 1 (AT1) receptor. [73]

This receptor called APJ had no known ligand until Tatemoto *et al* identified Apelin, a 36-AA peptide isolated from bovine stomach extracts that selectively binds to it. [74] Despite a high homology between APJ and AT1 receptors, Apelin does not bind to AT1 and Angiotensin has no affinity for APJ.

The human gene coding for Apelin is located on chromosome 11 and encodes a 77-AA pre-propeptide which is cleaved into several isoforms of varying lengths (12, 13, 16, 17, 19 and 36). [74-75] Plasma concentrations of the cleaved peptides range from 3 to 4 ng/ml which is a low concentration relative to other circulating hormones. [76] The shorter isoforms seem to exhibit the strongest activity, especially in the cardiovascular system. Apelin-APJ genes are ubiquitously expressed in the central nervous system (CNS), vascular endothelium, placenta, smooth muscle, mammary gland, kidney, lung, heart, and in several species including human. [77-78] The APJ receptor is expressed in heart myocytes and endothelium of large vessels, veins and arteries at a similar density to AT1 receptors. [79] The distribution of Apelin-APJ system in heart suggests that it is involved in vascular tone regulation, cardiac contraction and fluid homeostasis, and suggest that it may have a therapeutic effect in the treatment of heart failure. The role of the Apelin-APJ system in the cardiovascular system is closely related to the Renin-Angiotensin System (RAS) which acts through the Angiotensin II/AT receptor. The high homology between mRNA sequence of APJ and AT1 and the similarity in their distribution suggest that a cross talk with opposite effects exists between them. Several studies have pointed out some links between these two systems. The vasoconstrictive effect of the RAS system plays a key role in the pathogenesis of heart failure. It is currently thought that carboxypeptidase angiotensin converting enzyme (ACE) II which is involved in the degradation of Ang II into Ang [1-7] also cleaves Apelin-36 and -13 into inactive peptides (figure 1). [80-81] Moreover, Ishida *et al* showed that APJ knockout mice were more sensitive to low dose of Ang II compared to control mice thus suggesting that Apelin acts as a counter regulatory factor of the Ang II vasoconstrictive effect *in vivo.* [82] AT1 knockout mice have a lower resting systolic blood pressure than control mice due to the lack of Ang II. However, blood pressure is partially restored in the double knockout AT1/APJ mice reinforcing the concept that the Apelin-APJ is counter regulatory of the AT1-Ang II system *in vivo.* [83] The positive impacts of Apelin on heart failure injury are still unclear. However, it has been shown that Apelin-13 infusion during the first 20 minutes of reperfusion following ischemia is able to reduce the infarct size. [84] In humans, myocardial expression of Apelin, during autocrine/paracrine and/or autacoid activity, is increased during the early stage but decreases as disease progress.

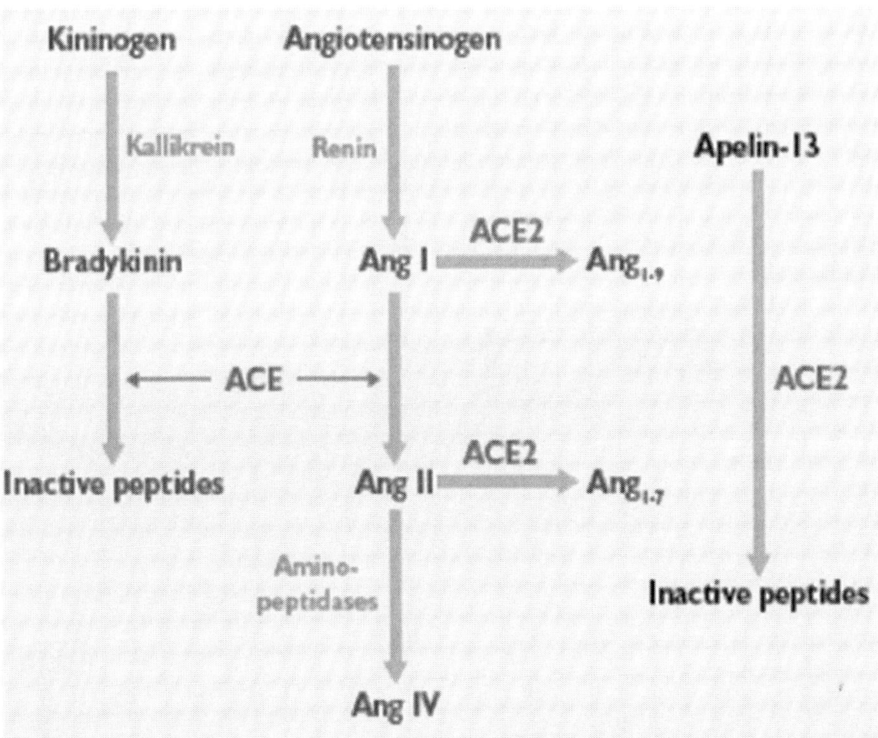

Figure 1. The renin-angiotensin-aldosterone system (RAAS). New component of RAAS, including Apelin, are shown in this model [85].

3. Apelin Regulates the Vascular Tone in a Nitric Oxide (NO) -Dependent Manner

Lee et al. found that intravenous (IV) infusion of Apelin-13 decreased both systolic and diastolic blood pressures in anaesthetized rats. [86] This reduction was inversely correlated to the molecular size of the different Apelin isoforms used and was abolished by NO synthase (NOS) inhibitor pre-treatment. [87] This result suggests that Apelin-induced vasodilatation is essentially NO-dependent. However, other studies showed that IV Apelin infusion can have a "paradoxal" vasoconstrictive effect. [88-89] Indeed, Tatemoto et al. found that the vasodilatatory effect of Apelin is endothelium-dependent and acts through Akt/eNOS activations, thus promoting NO release with increased GMPc levels. When the endothelium is dysfunctional, Apelin directly binds to the vascular smooth muscles APJ receptors and induces vasoconstriction (figure 2). Apelin can induce phosphorylation of the myosin light chain (MLC) in vascular smooth muscle cells that is necessary for the actin-myosin interaction and thus the MLC contraction (01). With or without a preserved endothelium, Apelin modulatory activity on contraction is of potential importance on systemic circulatory bed. It may also act on the lung low-pressure bed as this tissue expresses the highest level of Apelin/APJ receptors.

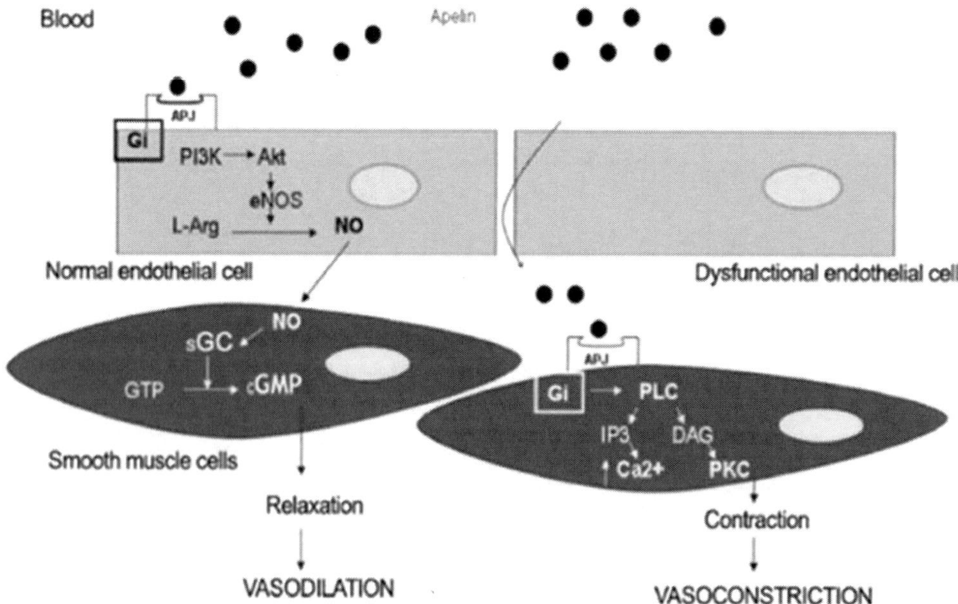

Figure 2. Intracellular pathways responsible for the vasomotor effects in the Apelin/APJ interaction in the absence and in the presence of endothelial dysfunction. DAG: Diaglycerol; eNOS: Endothelial Nitric Oxide Synthase; Gi: Inhibitory G protein; sGC: soluble Guanylate Cyclase; GTP: Guanosine Triphosphate; cGMP: Cyclic Guanosine Monophosphate; IP3: Inositol Triphosphate; L-Arg: L-Arginine; NCX: Na^{+}-Ca^{2+} Exchanger; NHE: Na^{+}-H^{+} Exchanger; NO: Nitric Oxide; PI3K: Phosphoinositide 3-kinase; PKC: Protein Kinase C; PLC: Phospholipase C [91].

4. Apelin Improves (Cardiac) Contractility

The APJ receptor is coupled with a Gi protein which is known to activate the phospholipase C (PLC) and protein kinase C (PKC). [92] The phosphorylation of the Na^+-H^+ exchanger (NHE) by PKC increases intracellular Na^+ resulting in enhanced intracellular Ca^{2+} by action of the reverse mode Na^+-Ca^{2+} exchanger (NCX). Cytosolic calcium is then more available and facilitates contraction (figure 3). Inhibiting PKC, PLC, NHE and NCX significantly blunts the positive inotropic effect of Apelin. [93] Apelin may also exert protective action on SR function and cardiac performance during ischemia-reperfusion by attenuating oxidation of SERCA and RyR. [94] Our group was among the first to show that APJ receptors are present in the cardiac ventricle of dogs where its activation by Apelin increases the amplitude of the sodium current (I_{NA}) and shifts its activation towards more negative potentials. The effects on I_{Na} were dependent on activation of PKC. The end result of these alterations is an increase in sodium entry and a reduction in the intra-extracellular sodium gradient that may increase contractility by reducing the turnover of the sodium-calcium and calcium extrusion during diastole (figure 3). These findings suggest that Apelin increases intracellular calcium concentrations and improves cardiac excitability. Such actions may prove beneficial in early phases of heart failure before loss of myofilament sensitivity to calcium and impairment of excitability.

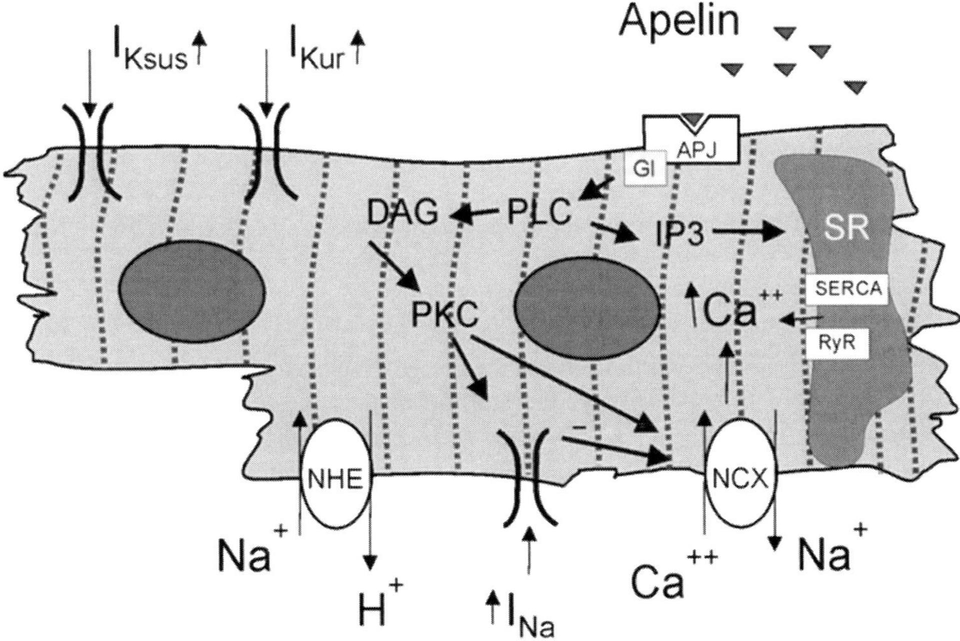

Figure 3. Intracellular pathways responsible for action potential modulation and positive inotropic effect of the Apelin/APJ interaction. $I_{Ksus,}$ I_{Kur}: Sustained and ultrarapid potassium currents (atrial); I_{Na}: cardiac sodium surrent DAG: Diaglycerol; Gi: Inhibitory G protein; IP3: Inositol Triphosphate; NCX: Na^+-Ca^{2+} Exchanger; NHE: Na^+-H^+ Exchanger; PKC: Protein Kinase C; PLC: Phospholipase C; SR: Sarcoplasmic Reticulum; SERCA: calcium ATPase pump; RyR ryanodine receptor, adapted from Ladeiras-Lopes et al., [91].

5. Apelin Has Protective Effects against Ischemic Heart Disease

Apelin plasma level plays a critical role by mitigating susceptibility to ischemic injuries and in functional recovery from ischemic heart failure. Reduced concentrations of circulating Apelin increase MI-related mortality, infarct size, and inflammation resulting in greater systolic dysfunction and heart failure [95] making it a potential therapeutic agent in ischemic heart disease.

This possibility is strongly supported by studies in dogs with microembolization-induced HF. In each animal receiving intravenous infusion, Apelin reduced end-diastolic volume (EDV), end-systolic volume (ESV) and increased left ventricular ejection fraction thus indicating that exogenous administration of Apelin improved LV systolic function even in advanced heart failure. [96]

In addition to previously mentioned effects on calcium regulation, recent evidence suggests that Apelin's protective effects against cardiac hypertrophy may also be linked to its ability to stimulate APJ receptors and confer resistance to chronic pressure overload. [97] Other results have shown that Apelin antagonizes cardiac impairment in sepsis by attenuating inflammatory responses suggesting a potential usefulness in sepsis and septic shock. [98]

6. Apelin Modulates Cardiac Electrical Activity

We have demonstrated that Apelin shifts the activation of the cardiac sodium current towards membrane potentials closer to the resting state. [99] This effect may therefore increase cardiac excitability.

In atrial cells, Apelin reduced action potential duration by up to 45% without changes in the amplitude or resting membrane potential. Apelin also increased the sodium current, ultra-rapid and sustained potassium currents and the reverse mode of sodium-calcium exchanger currents. Interestingly however, the late sodium currents and L-type calcium currents amplitudes were decreased and the authors did not observe changes in the transient outward currents or inward rectifier potassium currents in LA myocytes. [100]

These effects of Apelin on late I_{Na} and on I_{ca} will concur to reduce action potential duration. Overall, Apelin may therefore exert protective electrophysiological effects by increasing excitability of the cells and reducing action potential duration. Shorter action potential duration may also modulate intracellular calcium concentrations by altering sodium homeostasis and calcium entry into cardiomyocytes.

These effects may prove beneficial for reducing the risk of arrhythmias linked to calcium overloading and concurrently increase diastolic function in the early stages of heart failure. In agreement, low plasma Apelin levels have been proposed as an independent prognostic factor for arrhythmia recurrence in patients with atrial fibrillation treated with antiarrhythmic drugs and in identification of high-risk patients. [101]

7. Apelin Is Committed in the Cardiovascular Development and Angiogenesis [102-103]

Apelin-APJ system is present in embryonic and adult tissues. There is a high expression level of APJ receptor in the embryonic endothelium and retinal cells where Apelin induces the angiogenesis. In the early stages of the retinal angiogenesis APJ expression is increased until stabilization of the vessel formation. [104] Several studies support the idea that Apelin promotes endothelium cell proliferation at embryonic stages but also in some pathological conditions. The angiogenic effect of the Apelin could become an interesting feature for clinical usefulness. Agonists to APJ receptors in case of ischemia/infarcts may promote revascularization and enhance contractility, and antagonists may limit tumor growth. This idea is further supported by results showing that Apelin deficiency decreased vascular sprouting, impaired sprouting of human endothelial progenitor cells, and compromised in vivo myocardial angiogenesis. [95] Apelin also enhances cardiac differentiation of mouse and human ESCs [105-106], further establishing its role in cardiogenicity.

8. Apelin is a Modulator of Fluid Homeostasis

The mechanism by which Apelin contributes to fluid homeostasis is not fully understood but may involve the hypothalamus-aldosterone axis. The Apelin/APJ system is expressed in the hypothalamus and more precisely in the supraoptic and paraventricular areas.

This brain structure is known to be involved in fluid balance via antidiuretic hormone (ADH) production. There is controversial data coming from animal work in regards of the Apelin actions on ADH. O'Carroll et al. found that neurons expressing ADH mRNA also express Apelin receptor mRNA suggesting a regulation of the ADH release by Apelin. [107] Intra-cerebroventricular administration of Apelin-13 decreases the ADH circulating levels and improves water intake in rats. [108]

On the other side, Apelin/APG knockout mice did not show any differences in water intake and urinary electrolyte concentrations compared to controls. [82, 109] Even if contradictory, these observations raised important questions about the role of the Apelin/APJ system in fluid and cardiac homeostasis.

9. Apelin Exhibits Others Various Physiological Actions

In 2005, Boucher et al. found that Apelin is expressed and secreted by human and mouse adipocytes. [110] Plasma and adipocytes Apelin levels increase with obesity and glucose intolerance, suggesting a pathophysiological role in insulin resistance, obesity and type 2 diabetes. Insulin seems to increase Apelin expression. Physical activity and exercise increase Apelin-AJP expression in the cardiovascular system and reduce blood pressure levels in hypertensive individuals. [111] It seems that Apelin is also involved in immune signaling by modulation of T-cell activity in human cell lines and cytokine production in mice. [112-113]

Finally, APJ receptor acts as a co-receptor for the entry of HIV virus in host's cells and Apelin inhibits HIV viral entry into CD4+ and APJ+ cells proportionally to the Apelin isoform weight. [115-116].

More studies are required to resolve the unanswered questions about the exact role of the Apelin/APJ system and clarify several controversies present in the literature to determine the conditions in which the Apelin/APJ system is involved and its regulation.

However, its wide expression in many physiological mechanisms such as blood pressure regulation, myocardial protection and function optimization, interaction with the Ang II- AT1 system, modulation of cardiac muscle contraction-relaxation and its role in the pathogenesis of diseases with high morbidity and mortality levels throughout the world, make the Apelin/APJ system a future promising therapeutic target.

10. Apelin: A New Prospect for the Supportive Treatment of Sepsis-Induced Myocardial Dysfunction

Whereas potentially beneficial in heart failure as summarized in the figure 4, Apelin is also a promising candidate for future clinical applications in sepsis-induced myocardial dysfunction.

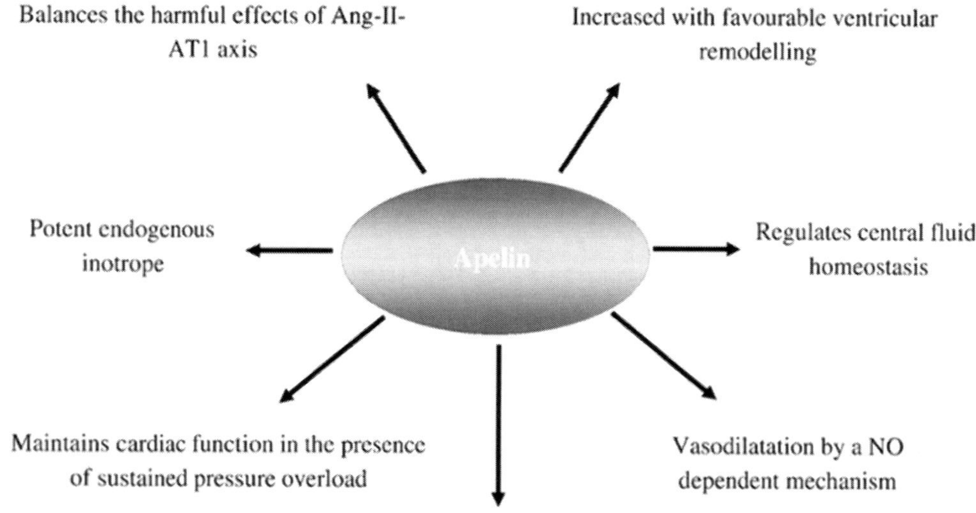

Figure 4. Summary of the various Apelin effects in heart failure. Ang II: Angiotensin II; AT1: Angiotensin II type 1 receptor; NO: Nitric Oxide [116].

Indeed, almost nothing is known as to Apelin's involvement in sepsis and its potential impact on outcome and induced myocardial dysfunction [117] but several specific impacts of Apelin draw inspirational avenues for future application of this molecule in sepsis . For instance, Apelin-related and cardiospecific effect can be ranged into a general protective property, while Apelin is known to prevent myocardial fibrosis/remodeling [118-119] and is directly committed in governing mesoderm patterning and cardiomyocyte specification [119] as well as to regulate progenitor cell trafficking. [120] Chronic Apelin-13 infusion inhibits monocyte-macrophage infiltration and related cytokine activities (including TNF-α expression) in aortic vascular wall, preventing aneurysm in an –induced model. [121] Blood level of Apelin is negatively correlated with C-reactive protein and Interleukin-6 blood in patients with end-stage renal failure. [122-123] Nonetheless, the links between the APL/APJ-R and NOS systems are well documented. [124] Inducible nitric oxide synthase (iNOS) increased expression in septic hearts is associated with myocardial dysfunction, and Apelin, through a NOS-dependent pathway, can improve heart function/recovery after induced ischemia [60,125-126], whereas Apelin-null mice exhibit a highly significant eNOS down-regulation. [127]

Apelin definitively has the potential to provide with a contractile added-value inside the myocardial tissue because transverse tubules and intercalated discs that originate at the Z-lines/bands are critical for cardiomyocyte homeostasis and water-solutes-energy exchanges; are essential to Ca^{2+} entry in the excitation-contraction processes [128], and the location where APJ-R is mainly expressed.

Preliminary data in our hands at the experimental level (i.e., a rat model of endotoxin-induced myocardial dysfunction) told us that Apelin exhibits similar inotropic impact than dobutamine in this context (figure 5). Further confirmatory studies will have to consolidate and refine these data in order to pave the way for subséquent phase I&II trials.

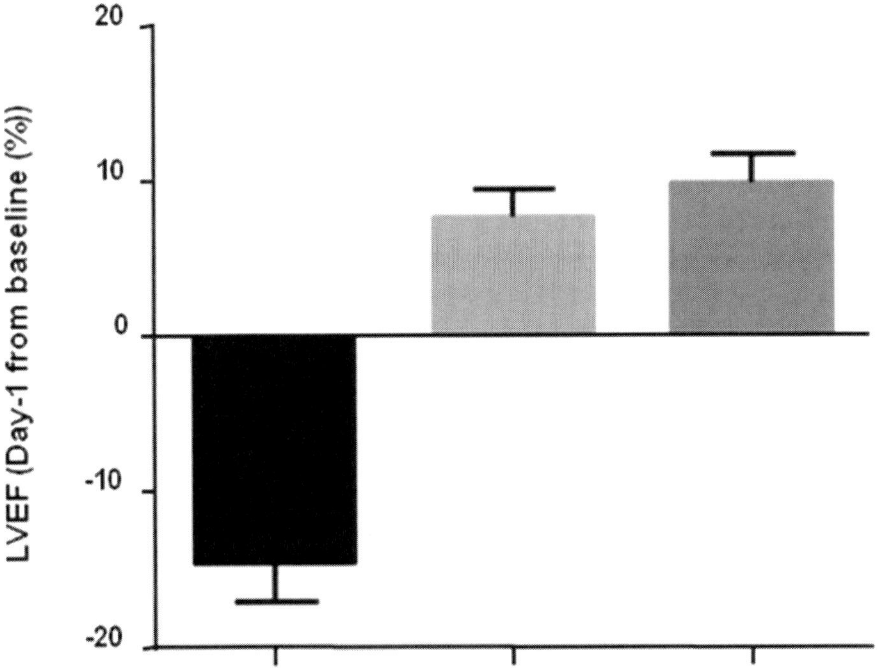

Figure 5. Modulation of Left Ventricular Ejection Fraction (LVEF) in rats injected with endotoxin (*E. Coli* lipopolysaccharides [LPS], 10mg/kg Intra/Peritoneal), and continuously infused (or not infused) with Intra/Venous (I/V) Apelin-13 peptide) or Dobutamine. ■ LPS; ■ LPS-Apelin-13 (0,25µg/kg/min I/V); ■ LPS-Dobutamine (7.5µg/kg/min I/V).

Conclusion

Apelin is a novel molecule with promising properties for therapeutic translation at bedside. Indeed, Apelin-APJ-R is another novel pathway by which efficient heart support can be provided to critically ill patients, especially those with severe sepsis or septic shock and myocardial impairment. Further clinical studies will allow to carve out more precise indications and safety issues for Apelin infusion, with forthcoming experimental evidence of efficiency.

References

[1] Gaieski DF, Edwards JM, Kallan MJ, Carr BG. Benchmarking the incidence and mortality of severe sepsis in the United States, *Crit Care Med,* 2013, 41: 1167-1174.

[2] Wenzel RP. Treating sepsis. *New Engl J Med,* 2002, 347: 966-7.

[3] Sands KE, Bates DW, Lanken PN, Graman PS, Hibberd PL, Kahn KL, Parsonnet J, Panzer R, Orav EJ, Snydman DR, Black E, Schwartz JS, Moore R, Johnson BL Jr, Platt R. Academic Medical Center Consortium Sepsis Project Working Group. Epidemiology of sepsis syndrome in 8 academic medical centers. *JAMA,* 1997, 278: 234-40.

[4] Rixen D, Siegel JH, Friedman HP. "Sepsis/SIRS," physiologic classification, severity stratification, relation to cytokine elaboration and outcome prediction in posttrauma critical illness. *J Trauma,* 1996, 41:581-98.

[5] Parrillo JE, Parker MM, Natanson C, Suffredini AF, Danner RL, Cunnion RE, Ognibene FP. Septic shock in humans. Advances in the understanding of pathogenesis, cardiovascular dysfunction, and therapy. *Ann Intern Med,* 1990, 113: 227-42.

[6] Vieillard-Baron A, Caille V, Charron C, Belliard G, Page B, Jardin F. Actual incidence of global left ventricular hypokinesia in adult septic shock. *Crit Care Med,* 2008, 36: 1701-6.

[7] Bouhemad B, Nicolas-Robin A, Arbelot C, Arthaud M, Féger F, Rouby JJ. Isolated and reversible impairment of ventricular relaxation in patients with septic shock. *Crit Care Med,* 2008, 36: 766-74.

[8] Bouhemad B, Nicolas-Robin A, Arbelot C, Arthaud M, Féger F, Rouby JJ. Acute left ventricular dilatation and shock-induced myocardial dysfunction. *Crit care Med,* 2009, 37: 441-7.

[9] Parker MM, Shelhamer JH, Bacharach SL, Green MV, Natanson C, Frederick TM, Damske BA, Parrillo JE. Profound but reversible myocardial depression in patients with septic shock. *An Intern Med,* 1984, 100: 483-90.

[10] Kumar A, Bunnell E, Lynn M, Anel R, Habet K, Neumann A, Parrillo JE. Experimental human endotoxemia is associated with depression of load-independent contractility indices: prevention by the lipid a analogue E5531. *Chest,* 2004, 126: 860-7.

[11] Dellinger RP, Levy MM, Rhodes A, Annane D, Gerlach H, Opal SM, Sevransky JE, Sprung CL, Douglas IS, Jaeschke R, Osborn TM, Nunnally ME, Townsend SR, Reinhart K, Kleinpell RN, Angus DC, Deutschman CS, Machado FR, Rubenfeld GD, Webb SA, Beale RJ, Vincent JL, Moreno R, and the Surviving Sepsis Campaign Guidelines Committee including the Pediatric Subgroup. Surviving Sepsis Campaign:

International Guidelines for Management of Severe Sepsis and Septic Shock: 2012. *Crit Care Med,* 2013, 41: 580-637.

[12] Kumar A, Schupp E, Bunnell E, Ali A, Milcarek B, Parrillo JE. Cardiovascular response to dobutamine stress predicts outcome in severe sepsis and septic shock. *Crit Care,* 2008, 12: R35.

[13] Vallet B, Chopin C, Curtis SE, Dupuis BA, Fourrier F, Mehdaoui H, LeRoy B, Rime A, Santre C, Herbecq P. Prognostic value of the dobutamine test in patients with sepsis syndrome and normal lactate values: a prospective, multicenter study. *Crit Care Med,* 1993, 21: 1868-75.

[14] Cunnion RE, Schaer GL, Parker MM, Natanson C, Parrillo JE. The coronary circulation in human septic shock. *Circulation,* 1986, 73: 637-44.

[15] Dhainaut JF, Huyghebaert MF, Monsallier JF, Lefevre G, Dall'Ava-Santucci J, Brunet F, Villemant D, Carli A, Raichvarg D. Coronary hemodynamics and myocardial metabolism of lactate, free fatty acids, glucose, and ketones in patients with septic shock. *Circulation,* 1987, 75: 533-41.

[16] Mehta S, Granton J, Gordon AC, Cook DJ, Lapinsky S, Newton G, Bandayrel K, Little A, Siau C, Ayers D, Singer J, Lee TCK, Walley KR, Storms M, Cooper DJ, Holmes CL, Hebert P, Presneill J, Russell JA for the VASST Investigators. Cardiac ischemia in patients with septic shock randomized to vasopressin or norepinephrine. *Crit Care,* 2013, 17: R117.

[17] Yu P, Boughner DR, Sibbald WJ, keys J, Dunmore J, Martin CM. Myocardial collagen changes and edema in rats with hyperdynamic sepsis. *Crit Care Med,* 1997, 25: 657-62.

[18] Quenot JP, Le Teuff G, Quantin C, Doise JM, Abrahamowicz M, Masson D, Blettery B. Myocardial injury in critically ill patients: relation to increased cardiac troponin I and hospital mortality. *Chest,* 2005, 128: 2758-64.

[19] Turner A, Tsamitros M, Bellomo R. Myocardial cell injury in septic shock. *Crit Care Med,* 1999, 27: 1775-80.

[20] Tavernier B, Li JM, El-Omar MM, Lanone S, Yang ZK, Trayer IP, Mebazaa A, Shah AM. Cardiac contractile impairment associated with increased phosphorylation of troponin I in endotoxemic rats. *FASEB J,* 2001, 15: 294-6.

[21] Flierl MA, Rittirsch D, Huber-Lang MS, Sarma JV, Ward PA. Molecular events in the cardiomyopathy of sepsis. *Mol Med,* 2008, 14: 327-36.

[22] Zernecke A, Bernhagen J, Weber C. Macrophage migration inhibitory factor in cardiovascular disease. *Circulation,* 2008, 117: 1594-602.

[23] Kapadia S, Lee J, Torre-Amione G, Birdsall HH, Ma TS, Mann DL. Tumor necrosis factor-alpha gene and protein expression in adult feline myocardium after endotoxin administration. *J Clin Invest*, 1995, 96: 1042-52.

[24] Fernandes CJ Jr, Akamine N, Knobel E. Myocardial depression in sepsis. *Shock,* 2008, 30, Suppl 1: 14-7.

[25] Goddard CM, Allard MF, Hogg JC, Herbertson MJ, Walley KR. Prolonged leukocyte transit time in coronary microcirculation of endotoxemic pigs. *Am J Physiol Heart,* 1995, 269: H1389-97.

[26] Granton JT, Goddard CM, Allard MF, van Eeden S, Walley KR. Leukocytes and decreased left-ventricular contractility during endotoxemia in rabbits. *Am J Respir Crit Care Med,* 1997, 155: 1977-83.

[27] Rossi MA, Celes MR, Prado CM, Saggioro FP. Myocardial structural changes in long-term human severe sepsis/septic shock may be responsible for cardiac dysfunction. *Shock,* 2007, 27: 10-8.

[28] dos Santos CC, Gattas DJ, Tsoporis JN, Smeding L, Kabir G, Masoom H, Akram A, Plotz F, Slutsky AS, Husain M, Sibbald WJ, Parker TG. Sepsis-induced myocardial depression is associated with transcriptional changes in energy metabolism and contractile related genes: a physiological and gene expression-based approach. *Crit Care Med,* 2010, 38: 894-902.

[29] Bianchi C, Araujo EG, Sato K, Sellke FW. Biochemical and structural evidence for pig myocardium adherens junction disruption by cardiopulmonary bypass. *Circulation,* 2001, 104 (Suppl 1): I319-24.

[30] Garner LB, Willis MS, Carlson DL, DiMaio JM, White MD, White DJ, Adams GA 4th, Horton JW, Giroir BP. Macrophage migration inhibitory factor is a cardiac-derived myocardial depressant factor. *Am J Physiol Heart Circ Physiol,* 2003, 285: H2500-9.

[31] Chagnon F, Metz C , Bucala R, Lesur O. MIF neutralizing can reverse myocardial dysfunction in endotoxinic shock. *Circulation Res,* 2005, 96: 1095 -1102.

[32] Matsui Y, Okamoto H, Jia N, Akino M, Uede T, Kitabatake A, Nishihira J. Blockade of macrophage migration inhibitory factor ameliorates experimental autoimmune myocarditis. *J Mol Cell Cardiol,* 2004, 37: 557-66.

[33] Lin X, Sakuragi T, Metz CN, Ojamaa K, Skopicki HA, Wang P, Al-Abed Y, Miller EJ. Macrophage migration inhibitory factor within the alveolar spaces induces changes in the heart during late experimental sepsis. *Shock,* 2005, 24: 556-63.

[34] Mezzani A, Corrà U, Giannuzzi P. Central adaptations to exercise training in patients with chronic heart failure. *Heart Fail Rev,* 2008, 13: 13-20.

[35] Friedrich MG. Myocardial edema--a new clinical entity? *Nature Rev Cardiol,* 2010, 7: 292-6

[36] Kellman P, Aletras AH, Mancini C, McVeigh ER, Arai AE. T2-prepared SSFP improves diagnostic confidence in edema imaging in acute myocardial infarction compared to turbo spin echo. *Magn Res Med* 2007, 57: 891-7.

[37] van den Berg BM, Vink H, Spaan JA. The endothelial glycocalyx protects against myocardial edema. *Circ Res,* 2003, 92: 592-4.

[38] Mehlhorn U, Geissler HJ, Laine GA, Allen SJ. Myocardial fluid balance. *Eur J CardioThor Surg,* 2001, 20: 1220-30.

[39] Ekerbicer N, Inan S, Tarakci F, Cilaker S, Ozbek M. Histophysiological effects of fluid resuscitation on heart, lung and brain tissues in rats with hypovolemia. *Acta Histochemica,* 2006, 108: 373-83.

[40] Deng X, Wang X, Andersson R. Endothelial barrier resistance in multiple organs after septic and nonseptic challenges in the rat. *J Appl Physiol,* 1995, 78: 2052-61.

[41] Gotloib L, Shostak A, Galdi P, Jaichenko J, Fudin R. Loss of microvascular negative charges accompanied by interstitial edema in septic rats' heart. *Circ Shock,* 1992, 36: 45-56.

[42] Au CG, Cooper ST, Lo HP, Compton AG, Yang N, Wintour EM, North KN, Winlaw DS. Expression of aquaporin 1 in human cardiac and skeletal muscle. *J Mol Cell Cardiol,* 2004, 36: 655-62.

[43] Birkenkamp-Demtroeder K, Bongartz S, Gams E, Kupfer C, Schipke JD, Schmitt M Expression of Water Channels in the Human Heart. *J Clin Basic Cardiol,* 2003, 6: 77-79.

[44] Jonker S, Davis LE, van der Bilt JD, Hadder B, Hohimer AR, Giraud GD, Thornburg KL. Anaemia stimulates aquaporin 1 expression in the fetal sheep heart. *Exp Physiol,* 2003, 88: 691-8.

[45] Egan JR, Butler TL, Cole AD, Abraham S, Murala JS, Baines D, Street N, Thompson L, Biecker O, Dittmer J, Cooper S, Au CG, North KN, Winlaw DS. Myocardial membrane injury in pediatric cardiac surgery: An animal model. *J Thor Cardiovasc Surg,* 2009, 137: 1154-62.

[46] Kuboshima S, Ogimoto G, Sakurada T, Fujino T, Sato T, Yasuda T, Maeba T, Owada S, Ishida M. Hyperosmotic stimuli induces recruitment of aquaporin-1 to plasma membrane in cultured rat peritoneal mesothelial cells. *Adv Perit Dial,* 2001, 17: 47-52.

[47] Okada Y, Maeno E. Apoptosis, cell volume regulation and volume-regulatory chloride channels. *Compar Biochem Physiol,* 2001, 130: 377-83.

[48] Baumgarten CM, Clemo HF. Swelling-activated chloride channels in cardiac physiology and pathophysiology. *Progress in Biophys & Mol Biol,* 2003, 82: 25-42.

[49] Chen CC, Lin YC, Chen SA, Luk HN, Ding PY, Chang MS, Chiang CE. Shortening of cardiac action potentials in endotoxic shock in guinea pigs is caused by an increase in nitric oxide activity and activation of the adenosine triphosphate-sensitive potassium channel. *Crit Care Med* 2000, 28: 1713-20.

[50] Chiang CE, Luk HN, Wang TM. Swelling-activated chloride current is activated in guinea pig cardiomyocytes from endotoxic shock. *Cardiovasc Res,* 2004, 62: 96-104.

[51] Yanagi N, Maruyama T, Arita M, Kaji Y, Niho Y. Alterations in electrical and mechanical activity in Langendorff-perfused guinea pig hearts exposed to decreased external sodium concentration with or without hypotonic insult. *Pathophysiol,* 2001, 7: 251-261.

[52] Thompson EB. Special topic: apoptosis. *Annu. Rev. Physiol,* 1998, 60: 525-32.

[53] Olivetti G, Abbi R, Quaini F, Kajstura J, Cheng W, Nitahara JA, Quaini E, Di Loreto C, Beltrami CA, Krajewski S, Reed JC, Anversa P. Apoptosis in the failing human heart. *N Engl J Med,* 1997, 336: 1131-41.

[54] Narula J, Kolodgie FD, Virmani R. Apoptosis and cardiomyopathy. *Current Opinion in Cardiol,* 2000, 15: 183-8.

[55] Dhanantwari P, Nadaraj S, Kenessey A, Chowdhury D, Al-Abed Y, Miller EJ, Ojamaa K. Macrophage migration inhibitory factor induces cardiomyocyte apoptosis. *Biochem Biophys Res Com,* 2008, 371: 298-303.

[56] Gill C, Mestril R, Samali A. Losing heart: the role of apoptosis in heart disease--a novel therapeutic target. *FASEB J,* 2002, 16: 135-46.

[57] Comstock KL, Krown KA, Page MT, Martin D, Ho P, Pedraza M, Castro EN, Nakajima N, Glembotski CC, Quintana PJ, Sabbadini RA. LPS-induced TNF-alpha release from and apoptosis in rat cardiomyocytes: obligatory role for CD14 in mediating the LPS response. *J Mol Cell Cardiol* 1998 30: 2761-75.

[58] Sugano M, Tsuchida K, Hata T, Makino N. In vivo transfer of soluble TNF-alpha receptor 1 gene improves cardiac function and reduces infarct size after myocardial infarction in rats. *FASEB J,* 2004, 18: 911-3.

[59] Raeburn CD, Calkins CM, Zimmerman MA, Song Y, Ao L, Banerjee A, Meng X, Harken AH. Vascular cell adhesion molecule--1 expression is obligatory for endotoxin-induced myocardial neutrophil accumulation and contractile dysfunction. *Surgery,* 2001, 130: 319-25.

[60] Walley KR, McDonald TE, Wang Y, Dai S, Russell JA. Albumin resuscitation increases cardiomyocyte contractility and decreases nitric oxide synthase II expression in rat endotoxemia. *Crit Care Med,* 2003, 31: 187-94.

[61] Lancel S, Petillot P, Favory R, Stebach N, Lahorte C, Danze PM, Vallet B, Marchetti P, Neviere R. Expression of apoptosis regulatory factors during myocardial dysfunction in endotoxemic rats. *Crit Care Med* 2005, 33: 492-6.

[62] McDonald TE, Grinman MN, Carthy CM, Walley KR. Endotoxin infusion in rats induces apoptotic and survival pathways in hearts. *Am J Physiol* (HCP), 2000, 279: H2053-61.

[63] Tanaka M, Nakae S, Terry RD, Mokhtari GK, Gunawan F, Balsam LB, Kaneda H, Kofidis T, Tsao PS, Robbins RC. Cardiomyocyte-specific Bcl-2 overexpression attenuates ischemia-reperfusion injury, immune response during acute rejection, and graft coronary artery disease. *Blood,* 2004, 104: 3789-96.

[64] Green DR. Apoptotic pathways: the roads to ruin. *Cell,* 1998, 94: 695-8.

[65] Balligand JL & Cannon PJ. In Contemporary cardiology, 4: NO and the cardiovascular system. Ed J Loscalzo et JA Vita, 2000. *Humana Press* Inc NJ.

[66] Agnoletti L, Curello S, Bachetti T, Malacarne F, Gaia G, Comini L, Volterrani M, Bonetti P, Parrinello G, Cadei M, Grigolato PG, Ferrari R. Serum from patients with severe heart failure downregulates eNOS and is proapoptotic: role of tumor necrosis factor-alpha. *Circulation,* 1999, 100: 1983-91.

[67] Burger D, Lei M, Geoghegan-Morphet N, Lu X, Xenocostas A, Feng Q. Erythropoietin protects cardiomyocytes from apoptosis via up-regulation of endothelial nitric oxide synthase. *Cardiovasc Res,* 2006, 72: 51-9.

[68] McKinnon RL, Lidington D, Bolon M, Ouellette Y, Kidder GM, Tyml K. Reduced arteriolar conducted vasoconstriction in septic mouse cremaster muscle is mediated by nNOS-derived NO. *Cardiovasc Res,* 2006, 69: 236-44.

[69] Lidington D, Li F, Tyml K. Deletion of neuronal NOS prevents impaired vasodilation in septic mouse skeletal muscle. *Cardiovasc Res* 2007, 74: 151-8.

[70] Martin SR, Emanuel K, Sears CE, Zhang YH, Casadei B. Are myocardial eNOS and nNOS involved in the beta-adrenergic and muscarinic regulation of inotropy? A systematic investigation. *Cardiovasc Res,* 2006, 70: 97-106.

[71] Geoghegan-Morphet N, Burger D, Lu X, Sathish V, Peng T, Sims SM, Feng Q. Role of neuronal nitric oxide synthase in lipopolysaccharide-induced tumor necrosis factor-alpha expression in neonatal mouse cardiomyocytes. *Cardiovasc Res,* 2007, 75: 408-16.

[72] Xu KY, Huso DL, Dawson TM, Bredt DS, Becker LC. Nitric oxide synthase in cardiac sarcoplasmic reticulum. *PNAS,* 1999, 96: 657-62.

[73] O'Dowd BF, Heiber M, Chan A, Heng HH, Tsui LC, Kennedy JL, Shi X, Petronis A, George SR, Nguyen T. A human gene that shows identity with the gene encoding the angiotensin receptor is located on chromosome 11. *Gene* 1993, 136(1-2):355-60.

[74] Tatemoto K, Hosoya M, Habata Y, Fujii R, Kakegawa T, Zou MX, Kawamata Y, Fukusumi S, Hinuma S, Kitada C, Kurokawa T, Onda H, Fujino M. Isolation and characterization of a novel endogenous peptide ligand for the human APJ receptor. *Biochem. Biophys. Res. Commun* 1998, 251, 471-6.

[75] Ali RH, Zareba W, Moss AJ, Schwartz PJ, Benhorin J, Vincent GM, Locati EH, Priori S, Napolitano C, Towbin JA, Hall WJ, Robinson JL, Andrews ML, Zhang L, Timothy K, Medina A. Clinical and genetic variables associated with acute arousal and nonarousal-related cardiac events among subjects with long QT syndrome. *Am J Cardiol* 2000, 85:457-61.

[76] Edinger AL, Hoffman TL, Sharron M, Lee B, Yi Y, Choe W, Kolson DL, Mitrovic B, Zhou Y, Faulds D, Collman RG, Hesselgesser J, Horuk R, Doms RW. An orphan seven-transmembrane domain receptor expressed widely in the brain functions as a coreceptor for human immunodeficiency virus type 1 and simian immunodeficiency virus. *J. Virol,* 1998, 72: 7934-40.

[77] Chamberland C, Barajas-Martinez H, Haufe V, Fecteau MH, Delabre JF, Burashnikov A, Antzelevitch C, Lesur O, Chraibi A, Sarret P, Dumaine R. Modulation of canine cardiac sodium current by Apelin. *J Mol. Cell Cardiol,* 2010, 48: 694-701.

[78] Kawamata Y, Habata Y, Fukusumi S, Hosoya M, Fujii R, Hinuma S, Nishizawa N, Kitada C, Onda H, Nishimura O, Fujino M. Molecular properties of apelin: tissue distribution and receptor binding. *Biochim. Biophys. Acta,* 2001, 1538: 162-71.

[79] Kleinz MJ, Skepper JN, Davenport AP. Immunocytochemical localisation of the apelin receptor, APJ, to human cardiomyocytes, vascular smooth muscle and endothelial cells. *Regul. Pept,* 2005, 126: 233-40.

[80] Vickers C, Hales P, Kaushik V, Dick L, Gavin J, Tang J, Godbout K, Parsons T, Baronas E, Hsieh F, Acton S, Patane M, Nichols A, Tummino P. Hydrolysis of biological peptides by human angiotensin-converting enzyme-related carboxypeptidase. *J. Biol. Chem,* 2002, 277: 14838-43.

[81] Lee DK, Saldivia VR, Nguyen T, Cheng R, George SR, O'Dowd BF. Modification of the terminal residue of apelin-13 antagonizes its hypotensive action. *Endocrinology* 2005, 146: 231-6.

[82] Ishida J, Hashimoto T, Hashimoto Y, Nishiwaki S, Iguchi T, Harada S, Sugaya T, Matsuzaki H, Yamamoto R, Shiota N, Okunishi H, Kihara M, Umemura S, Sugiyama F, Yagami K, Kasuya Y, Mochizuki N, Fukamizu A. Regulatory roles for APJ, a seven-transmembrane receptor related to angiotensin-type 1 receptor in blood pressure in vivo. *J Biol. Chem,* 2004, 279: 26274-9.

[83] Iwanaga Y, Kihara Y, Takenaka H, Kita T. Down-regulation of cardiac apelin system in hypertrophied and failing hearts: Possible role of angiotensin II-angiotensin type 1 receptor system. *J Mol. Cell Cardiol,* 2006, 41: 798-806.

[84] Rastaldo R, Cappello S, Folino A, Berta GN, Sprio AE, Losano G, Samaja M, Pagliaro P. Apelin-13 limits infarct size and improves cardiac postischemic mechanical recovery only if given after ischemia. *Am. J Physiol Heart Circ,* 2011, 300: H2308-15.

[85] Quazi, R., C. Palaniswamy, W. H. Frishman. The emerging role of apelin in cardiovascular disease and health. *Cardiol. Rev,* 2009,17: 283-6.

[86] Lee DK, Cheng R, Nguyen T, Fan T, Kariyawasam AP, Liu Y, Osmond DH, George SR, O'Dowd BF. Characterization of apelin, the ligand for the APJ receptor. *J. Neurochem,* 2000, 74: 34-41.
[87] Tatemoto K, Takayama K, Zou MX, Kumaki I, Zhang W, Kumano K, Fujimiya M. The novel peptide apelin lowers blood pressure via a nitric oxide-dependent mechanism. *Regul. Pept,* 2001, 99: 87-92.
[88] Charles CJ, Rademaker MT, Richards AM. Apelin-13 induces a biphasic haemodynamic response and hormonal activation in normal conscious sheep. *J Endocrinol,* 2006, 189: 701-10.
[89] Seyedabadi M, Goodchild AK, Pilowsky PM. Site-specific effects of apelin-13 in the rat medulla oblongata on arterial pressure and respiration. *Auton. Neurosci,* 2002, 101: 32-8.
[90] Chiba K, Sugiyama A, Watanabe K, Takasuna K, Hashimoto K. Acute hypokalemia may not be an effective way to sensitize the in situ canine heart for sparfloxacin-induced long QT syndrome. *J Pharmacol,* 2006, 100: 88-92.
[91] Ladeiras-Lopes R, Ferreira-Martins J, Leite-Moreira AF, The apelinergic system: the role played in human physiology and pathology and potential therapeutic applications. *Arq Bras. Cardiol.* 2008, 90: 343-9.
[92] Falcao-Pires I, Leite-Moreira AF. Apelin: a novel neurohumoral modulator of the cardiovascular system. Pathophysiologic importance and potential use as a therapeutic target. *Rev. Port. Cardiol,* 2005, 24: 1263-76.
[93] Szokodi I, Tavi P, Földes G, Voutilainen-Myllylä S, Ilves M, Tokola H, Pikkarainen S, Piuhola J, Rysä J, Tóth M, Ruskoaho H. Apelin, the novel endogenous ligand of the orphan receptor APJ, regulates cardiac contractility. *Circ. Res.* 2002, 691: 434-40.
[94] Wang C, Liu N, Luan R, Li Y, Wang D, Zou W, Xing Y, Tao L, Cao F, Wang H. Apelin protects sarcoplasmic reticulum function and cardiac performance in ischaemia-reperfusion by attenuating oxidation of sarcoplasmic reticulum Ca2+-ATPase and ryanodine receptor. *Cardiovasc Res.* 2013 Jul 16. [Epub ahead of print]
[95] Wang W, McKinnie SM, Patel VB, Haddad G, Wang Z, Zhabyeyev P, Das SK, Basu R, McLean B, Kandalam V, Penninger JM, Kassiri Z, Vederas JC, Murray AG, Oudit GY. Loss of Apelin Exacerbates Myocardial Infarction Adverse Remodeling and Ischemia-reperfusion Injury: Therapeutic Potential of Synthetic Apelin Analogues. *J Am. Heart Assoc,* 2013, 2: e000249.
[96] Wang M, Gupta RC, Rastogi S, Kohli S, Sabbah MS, Zhang K, Mohyi P, Hogie M, Fischer Y, Sabbah HN. Effects of acute intravenous infusion of apelin on left ventricular function in dogs with advanced heart failure. *J Card Fail,* 2013, 19: 509-16.
[97] Scimia MC, Hurtado C, Ray S, Metzler S, Wei K, Wang J, Woods CE, Purcell NH, Catalucci D, Akasaka T, Bueno OF, Vlasuk GP, Kaliman P, Bodmer R, Smith LH, Ashley E, Mercola M, Brown JH, Ruiz-Lozano P. APJ acts as a dual receptor in cardiac hypertrophy. *Nature,* 2012, 488: 394-8.
[98] Pan CS, Teng X, Zhang J, Cai Y, Zhao J, Wu W, Wang X, Tang CS, Qi YF. Apelin antagonizes myocardial impairment in sepsis. *J Card Fail,* 2010, 16: 609-17.
[99] Chamberland C, Barajas-Martinez H, Haufe V, Fecteau MH, Delabre JF, Burashnikov A, Antzelevitch C, Lesur O, Chraibi A, Sarret P, Dumaine R. Modulation of canine cardiac sodium current by Apelin. *J Mol. Cell Cardiol,* 2010, 48: 694-701.

[100] Cheng CC, Weerateerangkul P, Lu YY, Chen YC, Lin YK, Chen SA, Chen YJ. Apelin regulates the electrophysiological characteristics of atrial myocytes. *Eur. J Clin. Invest, 2013*, 43, 34-40.

[101] Falcone C, Buzzi MP, D'Angelo A, Schirinzi S, Falcone R, Rordorf R, Capettini AC, Landolina M, Storti C, Pelissero G. Apelin plasma levels predict arrhythmia recurrence in patients with persistent atrial fibrillation. *Int. J Immunopathol. Pharmacol,* 2010, 23: 917-25.

[102] Zeng XX, Wilm TP, Sepich DS, Solnica-Krezel L. Apelin and its receptor control heart field formation during zebrafish gastrulation. *Dev. Cell,* 2007, 12: 391-402.

[103] Kasai A, Shintani N, Oda M, Kakuda M, Hashimoto H, Matsuda T, Hinuma S, Baba A. Apelin is a novel angiogenic factor in retinal endothelial cells. *Biochem. Biophys. Res Commun,* 2004, 325: 395-400.

[104] Saint-Geniez M, Argence CB, Knibiehler B, Audigier Y. The msr/apj gene encoding the apelin receptor is an early and specific marker of the venous phenotype in the retinal vasculature. *Gene Expr. Patterns,* 2003, 3: 467-72.

[105] Wang IN, Wang X, Ge X, Anderson J, Ho M, Ashley E, Liu J, Butte MJ, Yazawa M, Dolmetsch RE, Quertermous T, Yang PC. Apelin enhances directed cardiac differentiation of mouse and human embryonic stem cells. *PLoS. One,* 2012, 7: e38328.

[106] Gao LR, Zhang NK, Bai J, Ding QA, Wang ZG, Zhu ZM, Fei YX, Yang Y, Xu RY, Chen Y. The apelin-APJ pathway exists in cardiomyogenic cells derived from mesenchymal stem cells in vitro and in vivo. *Cell Transplant,* 2010, 19: 949-58.

[107] O'Carroll AM, Don AL, Lolait SJ. APJ receptor mRNA expression in the rat hypothalamic paraventricular nucleus: regulation by stress and glucocorticoids. Regulation of rat APJ receptor messenger ribonucleic acid expression in magnocellular neurones of the paraventricular and supraopric nuclei by osmotic stimuli. *J Neuroendocrinol*, 2003,15: 1095-101.

[108] Taheri S, Murphy K, Cohen M, Sujkovic E, Kennedy A, Dhillo W, Dakin C, Sajedi A, Ghatei M, Bloom S. The effects of centrally administered apelin-13 on food intake, water intake and pituitary hormone release in rats. *Biochem. Biophys. Res Commun,* 2002, 291: 1208-12.

[109] Kuba K, Zhang L, Imai Y, Arab S, Chen M, Maekawa Y, Leschnik M, Leibbrandt A, Markovic M, Schwaighofer J, Beetz N, Musialek R, Neely GG, Komnenovic V, Kolm U, Metzler B, Ricci R, Hara H, Meixner A, Nghiem M, Chen X, Dawood F, Wong KM, Sarao R, Cukerman E, Kimura A, Hein L, Thalhammer J, Liu PP, Penninger JM. Impaired heart contractility in Apelin gene-deficient mice associated with aging and pressure overload. *Circ. Res,* 2007, 101: 32-42.

[110] Boucher J, Masri B, Daviaud D, Gesta S, Guigné C, Mazzucotelli A, Castan-Laurell I, Tack I, Knibiehler B, Carpéné C, Audigier Y, Saulnier-Blache JS, Valet P. Apelin, a newly identified adipokine up-regulated by insulin and obesity. *Endocrinology,* 2005, 146: 1764-71.

[111] Jia YX, Pan CS, Zhang J, Geng B, Zhao J, Gerns H, Yang J, Chang JK, Tang CS, Qi YF. Apelin protects myocardial injury induced by isoproterenol in rats. *Regul. Pept.* 2006, 133: 147-54.

[112] Y. Horiuchi, T. Fujii, Y. Kamimura, K. Kawashima. The endogenous, immunologically active peptide apelin inhibits lymphocytic cholinergic activity during immunological responses. *J Neuroimmunol,* 2003, 144: 46-52.

[113] Habata Y, Fujii R, Hosoya M, Fukusumi S, Kawamata Y, Hinuma S, Kitada C, Nishizawa N, Murosaki S, Kurokawa T, Onda H, Tatemoto K, Fujino M. Apelin, the natural ligand of the orphan receptor APJ, is abundantly secreted in the colostrum. *Biochim. Biophys*, 1999,1452: 25-35.

[114] Cayabyab M, Hinuma S, Farzan M, Choe H, Fukusumi S, Kitada C, Nishizawa N, Hosoya M, Nishimura O, Messele T, Pollakis G, Goudsmit J, Fujino M, Sodroski J. Apelin, the natural ligand of the orphan seven-transmembrane receptor APJ, inhibits human immunodeficiency virus type 1 entry. *J Virol,* 2000, 74: 11972-6.

[115] Zou MX, Liu HY, Haraguchi Y, Soda Y, Tatemoto K, Hoshino H. Apelin peptides block the entry of human immunodeficiency virus (HIV). *FEBS Lett,* 2000, 473: 15-8.

[116] Chandrasekaran B, Dar O, McDonagh T. The role of apelin in cardiovascular function and heart failure. *Eur. J Heart Fail,* 2008, 10: 725-32.

[117] Lesur O, Roussy JF, Chagnon F, Gallo-Payet N, Dumaine R, Sarret P, Chraibi A, Chouinard L, Hoge B. Proven infection-related sepsis induces a differential stress response early after ICU admission. *Crit Care,* 2010, 14: R131.

[118] Siddiquee K, Hampton J, Khan S, Zadory D, Gleaves L, Vaughan DE, Smith LH. Apelin protects against angiotensin II-induced cardiovascular fibrosis and decreases plasminogen activator inhibitor type-1 production. *J Hypertension,* 2011, 29: 724-31.

[119] Falcão-Pires I, Gonçalves N, Henriques-Coelho T, Moreira-Gonçalves D, Roncon-Albuquerque R Jr, Leite-Moreira AF. Apelin decreases myocardial injury and improves right ventricular function in monocrotaline-induced pulmonary hypertension. *Am J Physiol Heart,* 2009, 296: H2007-14.

[120] D'Aniello C, Lonardo E, Iaconis S, Guardiola O, Liguoro AM, Liguori GL, Autiero M, Carmeliet P, Minchiotti G. G protein-coupled receptor APJ and its ligand apelin act downstream of Cripto to specify embryonic stem cells toward the cardiac lineage through extracellular signal-regulated kinase/p70S6 kinase signaling pathway. *Circ Res,* 2009, 105: 231-8.

[121] Leeper NJ, Tedesco MM, Kojima Y, Schultz GM, Kundu RK, Ashley EA, Tsao PS, Dalman RL, Quertermous T. Apelin prevents aortic aneurysm formation by inhibiting macrophage inflammation. *Am J Physiol Heart,* 2009, 296: H1329-35.

[122] El-Shehaby AM, Zakaria A, El-Khatib M, Mostafa N. Association of fetuin-A and cardiac calcification and inflammation levels in hemodialysis patients. *Scand J Clin & Lab Invest,* 2010, 70: 575-82.

[123] Ashley E, Chun HJ, Quertermous T. Opposing cardiovascular roles for the angiotensin and apelin signaling pathways. *J Mol Cell Cardiol,* 2006, 41: 778-81.

[124] Ishida J, Hashimoto T, Hashimoto Y, Nishiwaki S, Iguchi T, Harada S, Sugaya T, Matsuzaki H, Yamamoto R, Shiota N, Okunishi H, Kihara M, Umemura S, Sugiyama F, Yagami K, Kasuya Y, Mochizuki N, Fukamizu A. Regulatory roles for APJ, a seven-transmembrane receptor related to angiotensin-type 1 receptor in blood pressure in vivo. *J Biol Chem,* 2004, 279: 26274-9.

[125] Rastaldo R, Cappello S, Folino A, Berta GN, Sprio AE, Losano G, Samaja M, Pagliaro P. Apelin-13 limits infarct size and improves cardiac postischemic mechanical recovery only if given after ischemia. *Am J Physiol Heart,* 2011, 300: H2308-15.
[126] Tamion F, Bauer F, Richard V, Laude K, Renet S, Slama M, Thuillez C. Myocardial dysfunction in early state of endotoxemia role of heme-oxygenase-1. *J Surg Res,* 2010, 158: 94-103.
[127] Chandra SM, Razavi H, Kim J, Agrawal R, Kundu RK, de Jesus Perez V, Zamanian RT, Quertermous T, Chun HJ. Disruption of the apelin-APJ system worsens hypoxia-induced pulmonary hypertension. *Arterioscler Thromb Vasc Biol,* 2011, 31: 814-20.
[128] Miller RT. Aquaporin in the heart--only for water? *J Mol Cell Cardiol,* 2004, 36: 653-4.

In: Sepsis
Editor: Nancy Khardori

ISBN: 978-1-63117-244-1

Chapter 3

Acute Kidney Injury in Sepsis

Marcelo Rodrigues Bacci, M.D.*
General Practice Department-Faculdade de Medicina do ABC
(ABC Medical School)- São Paulo- Brazil

Abstract

Sepsis and acute kidney injury (AKI) are two of the main causes of hospitalization in intensive care units (ICU) and account for a large proportion of deaths in these units in spite of continuous intense investigation at different levels. Sepsis is one of the leading cause of AKI. Understanding its pathophysiology was difficult in the past because of lack of data from study of kidney biopsies. Therefore, the so called "Acute Tubular Necrosis" did not fit in this scenario as sepsis-induced AKI is a major hemodynamic situation with an increase in blood flow and a decrease in filtration pressure. Also, there are non-hemodynamic factors that play an important role in sepsis- induced AKI. The cytokines like interleukin-6, interleukin-1, tumor necrosis factor-alpha act as potential stimulators of apoptosis, leukocyte activation and necrosis. Treatment of Sepsis-induced AKI is directed at controlling the arterial pressure, managing glycemia and using appropriate antimicrobial therapy. Specific substances to stop the process of AKI are not available l yet for human usage. Dialysis methods should be chosen based on patients' needs.

Keywords: Acute Kidney Injury, Sepsis, Tubular Cell Apoptosis, TNf-Alpha

Introduction

Sepsis and acute kidney injury (AKI) are two of the major causes of hospitalization in intensive care units (ICU) and account for a large proportion of deaths in these units. The diagnosis and management of sepsis have received intense investigation but the morbidity and

* Email: mrbacci@yahoo.com

mortality remain high. In one of the first reports on the extension of this serious health situation, in 2001, Angus et al. conducted an observational study using the current definition of sepsis and the 9thedition of the international code of diseases, revealing an alarming number on the average hospitalization days and expenses in dollars per patient. The average cost was US$ 22,100 per patient with an inpatient hospital time of 19.9 days [1]. Hall et al. conducted a survey of the number of hospitalizations due to sepsis or with the development of sepsis during the years 2001 to 2008. Using the National Hospital Discharge Survey they observed, as shown in Fig.1, an increase from 326,000 hospitalizations for septicemia or sepsis in 2000 to 727,000 in the year 2008 and with the rate of hospitalization for every 10,000 inhabitants doubling from 11.6% to 24% in the same period [2].

AKI in ICU is quite common and has very conflicting incidence data. Defining its incidence is difficult because of the large number of definitions of acute kidney injury in recent decades and eventually orienting the contemporary studies towards each one of these definitions. For example, depending on the definition used, this incidence ranged from 1% up to 70% [3]. Chertow and Bonventre in 2005 conducted a survey with demographic data and tracking number of requests for creatinine level and compared these with hospitalization time, cost and mortality in an intervention guided by computer data. They observed that approximately 30% of patients with at least three collections for creatinine level, obtained variations between 0.3 mg/dl and 0.4 mg/dl [4]. This data corresponded to about 70% more chance of death compared with those who had no oscillation of the value of creatinine, even when it was higher than 2 mg/dl. The National Center for Health Statistics in 2001 observed there were approximately 122 hospital discharged patients for every 1,000 patients not institutionalized, which corresponds to nearly 34,000,000 of admissions with AKI per year [4].

Using the current definitions, based on the value of elevated creatinine and urine output per unit of time, we found, 20% of hospitalized patients with acute kidney injury, in a general way and without division of its etiology in a series in 2012. [5] Separating by etiology, and considering only sepsis as a cause of acute kidney injury, we found that in patients with sepsis within 24 hours of the diagnosis, approximately 64.4% had already presented with acute kidney injury using the diagnostic criterion RIFLE [6].

Definitions

Sepsis is defined as the presence of Systemic Inflammatory Response Syndrome (SIRS) associated with an infectious focus (known or assumed) resulting in systemic effects [7, 8]. Severe sepsis is defined as the extension of previous sepsis which causes organ dysfunction and/or tissue hypoperfusion [8]. The definition of acute kidney injury has been the object of study in the last decades. The consensual current term, acute kidney injury, encompasses the occurrence of small changes, which were not captured due to the misuse of the term failure. However, the concept of injury involves the idea of tissue change, which is often not present [9].The renal function is analyzed by the variation of serum creatinine and urinary output. Urinary output less than 400 ml in 24h is defined as oliguria and less than 100 ml per day as anuria. The oscillations in the creatinine values remain the gold standard for classification of renal insult. `Two classifications in terms of urinary output per unit of weight and time and in terms of oscillation in basal value of creatinine are extremely important as they define the severity and the outcome of acute kidney injury.

Table 1 demonstrates the RIFLE classification, adopted by Acute Dialysis Quality Initiative (ADQI) where each letter represents a phase of the status of renal injury. R represents Risk, I injury, F failure, L loss and E end-stage renal disease. The first three statuses are based on changes in the values of serum creatinine and urine output and the last two on the of evolution time of renal failure [10].

Table 1. Rifle Classification

Stage	Creatinine and GFR Criteria	Urine Output Criteria
R- Risk	↓GFR 25% or ↑ SCr 50%	< 0.5 ml/kg/h for 6 hours
I- Injury	↓ GFR 50% or ↑SCr 100%	< 0.5 ml/kg/h for 12 hours
F- Failure	↓GFR 75% or ↑ SCr 200%	< 0.3 ml/kg/h for 24 hours or anuria for 12 hours
L- Loss	AKI for 4 weeks	
E- End Stage Renal Disease	Permanent dyalisis	

Table 2. Akin Classification

Stage	Creatinine and GFR Criteria	Urine Output Criteria
I	↑ SCr 50% or ↑ 0.3 mg/dl	< 0.5 ml/kg/h for 6 hours
II	↑ SCr 100%	< 0.5 ml/kg/h for 12 hours
III	↑ SCr 200%	< 0.3 ml/kg/h for 24 hours or anuria for 12 hours

Table 2 presents the AKIN classification, adopted by the National Kidney Foundation and disseminated by Kidney Disease Initiative: Improving Global Outcomes Clinical Practice Guideline for Acute Kidney Injury (KDIGO), which also is based on the oscillation of the value of the baseline serum creatinine and/or urinary output per unit of weight and time [11].Both classifications are similar and show concern for small oscillations in the creatinine value as evidence of renal injury. This observation has led to the likelyhood of the risk of diagnosing renal injury as any changes in the value of serum creatinine. The creatinine as an indicator of renal dysfunction is a late marker and is influenced by several factors such as drugs, ethnicity, sex, and muscle mass.

Markers of tubular injury by definition do not estimate the glomerular filtration rate, which is restricted to the measurement of serum creatinine and cystatin C, which is a non-glycosylated protein, produced constantly by all nucleated cells. Having low molecular weight, the cystatin C is freely filtered by the glomerulus and not secreted by tubule, serving as a good marker of glomerular filtration rate (GFR).The complexity of the patient with critical illness and multiple variables involved in its treatment hinder a homogenization of the population for the development of the model which adequately estimates glomerular filtration rate in patients with acute kidney injury.

The existing equations, Cockroft-Gault, MDRD, CKD-EPI, were based for stable patients and without AKI. Therefore, they do not have accuracy for routine use in critically ill patients [12-13].

Recently, Brugadotiir et al. compared the calculation of glomerular filtration rate by creatinine clearance by the three commonly used equations and to that by clearance of acid chromium-etilenodiaminicotetra-acetic (Cr-EDTA) [14]. They observed that, compared with the clearance of Cr-EDTA, the equations had performed poorly with error of 67.8% for the MDRD and 68.8% for the CKD-EPI. The error was 103% when the comparison was made with creatinine clearance [14].Models that estimate the glomerular filtration rate (GFR) in critically ill patients, as explained previously, are difficult to reproduce. To improve reproducibility, Chen used an algorithm and proposed an equation that appreciates the changes in creatinine values over the period of acute kidney injury, affecting not only the time of worsening but also the time of recovery of renal function. Although not validated, the existence of this model, the KeGFR (Kinect estimated GFR), seems promising [15].

Biomarkers of Renal Injury in Sepsis

As mentioned before, the prediction models of glomerular filtration rate are unreliable for patients with acute dysfunction which has led to the creation of classifications for stratification of acute kidney injury based on the variation in the value of creatinine and urine output.The creatinine is a late AKI biomarker with the limitations of a huge plasma volume distribution, extreme gender and body muscle content variability and also ethnic variability. However, creatinine is a low cost biomarker and easy to perform.

In general it is postulated that for every reduction by half in glomerular filtration rate the creatinine doubles in value. Nonetheless, the factors that determine its concentration such as the rate of production, volume of distribution and excretion rate, float causing delay in early detection of renal dysfunction. A good example of this limitation concerns the existence of positive hydric balance or accumulated one. Positive hydric balance is quite common in ICU patients because of the use of volume expansion bundle in the initial management of sepsis [16].

Contrary to what is commonly thought, the lower the creatinine in critically ill patients the worse is the outcome. This association exists because of the associated risk of fluid overload which retards the creatinine increase thus delaying the diagnosis of AKI and the measures for its reversal16.Cerda et al. have shown a better outcome in patients with higher serum creatinine levels. As the volume of distribution of liquids is increased in these patients, the same happens to the distribution of serum creatinine which reduces the sensitivity of detecting the increase of its value [17].

The cystatin C is a protein of low molecular weight, 16 KDa, produced by all nucleated cells. By having low molecular weight, it has free passage by glomerulus and is reabsorbed by proximal convoluted tubule, but without being secreted by the kidney or any other extra-renal structure. It also presents anthropometric and gender influences, but of a smaller magnitude than the creatinine. The time sequence of its rise after development of AKI is controversial and the reports differ. In a model of cardiac surgery in adults its serial elevation occurred 6 hours after the procedure with a specificity of 86% [18]. Another study using a mixed population of critically ill patients, reported that the cystatin C diagnosed acute kidney injury approximately 1.5 days earlier that the creatinine [19].A recent cohort study compared the sensitivity of cystatin C to estimate GFR with creatinine and its correlation with cardiovascular outcomes. Higher cystatin C levels were correlated with worse cardiovascular outcomes, mortality and chronic kidney disease staging. Despite this strong association, this population did not have AKI [20].

Interleukin 18 (IL18) is an acute-phase protein of low molecular weight and is produced by cleavage of caspase. It acts as an inflammation modulating protein and has elevated urinary levels in processes of ischemia and reperfusion. Its role in sepsis is still controversial [21]. The lipocalin associated with human neutrophil gelatinase (NGAL) is a protein with molecular weight of 25 KDa, which is synthesized and secreted by proximal tubular and distal cells and freely filtered by the glomerulus. In healthy kidneys its levels are hardly detectable. However, in the presence of acute tubular injury, its serum and urinary levels become quite high. In a model of cardiac surgery in children its elevation occurred 2 hours after establishment of the extracorporeal circulation with an area under the curve of 0.99 [22].

In adults these data are conflicting. The NGAL rise times vary from 2 to 18 hours after the installation of extracorporeal circulation [23]. This variation can be explained by the heterogeneity of comorbidities in these patients and therefore, questions its use in patients with prior alteration of renal function and/or with other etiologies for acute kidney injury, except the ischemicones [19].A recent meta-analysis showed that the NGAL is sensitive and specific in the early detection of renal pathology regardless of etiology (nephropathy by contrast, renal injury after surgery, sepsis). A limiting factor for the use of the NGAL in these studies is that its cut-off value was not well established and various definitions of acute kidney injury were used in several studies that comprised this meta-analysis [24].

NGAL presents distinct isomeric forms according to their place of production and may be elevated in sepsis without any development of AKI. Themonomeric form has a molecular weight of approximately 25kDa and it is released by neutrophils and renal tubular epithelium. The heterodimer form weighs approximately 135kDa and is exclusively released by the renal tubular epithelium. Small quantities in urine make its detection difficult. The homodimer form has a molecular weight of 45kDa and is released only by neutrophils [25]. Commercial kits for NGAL detection by ELISA do not distinguish isoforms which complicate the identification of the original production siteand its interpretation instates of sepsis [25].Doi et al. demonstrated that compared to other markers such as Interleukin18, NGAL was inferior in detecting AKI in the presence of sepsis. Instead, its rise was not associated with AKI according to AKIN and RIFLE criteria [26]. Despite that, NGAL serum levels are higher than creatinine in all conditions: children, adults, post-surgical and septic patients.

The KIM-1, acronym for Kidney Injury Molecule 1, is a Trans membrane glycoprotein found in apical edge of cells in the tubular epithelium in acute and chronic processes. It is not detectable in normal kidneys and it is believed that it may participate in the process of tubular regeneration [24]. Its functional role to detect acute kidney injury of septic origin is not well established yet [21].

Approximately 30% of patients with acute kidney injury in a recent observational series have chronic renal disease at admission. Serial determination of the levels of these markers can be crucial in determining whether it is pre-existing or new renal injury. However, the presence of prior proteinuria seems to increase the urinary levels of cystatin C and NGAL

[27].The joint use of biomarkers of glomerular filtration and structural change increases the sensitivity for early detection of acute kidney injury and determination of its cause.

Pathophysiology

Hemodynamic Factors

One of the most significant historical difficulties for understanding of the mechanism of sepsis induced acute kidney injury is the lack of renal biopsies in these patients. The clinical status and impediments arising from multiple comorbidities, such as hemodynamic instability, coagulopathies, prevent the routine performance and serial biopsies for histological analysis of the process and monitoring of its evolution.

In a systematic review, Langerbergh et al. observed only 6 septic AKI studies with renal biopsies. The 184 patients in this series revealed acute tubular necrosis in only 22% of patients. Therefore, 78% did not have the well-known mechanism of AKI [28]. Due to that difficulties in obtaining human data, animal models ware created and their concepts were applied to human body. However, the majority of animal models were made through injury from ischemia and reperfusion, which does not reflect what occurs in sepsis. This situation reflects what occurs in cases of hypodynamic shock as the cardiogenic, hypovolemic and possibly the septic one, depending on its phase.

However, in the hyperdynamic and septic model in pigs, as Ravikant et al. showed [25], an increase in both cortical and medullar renal blood flow occurs [29]. Measurements of renal blood flow via thermodilution catheters showed renal injury with increased or normal blood flow [30]. This observation is most of the times found in humans, a model in hyperdynamic sepsis. This is the main reason for different results in many experimental studies due to differences in physiological behavior in relation to the type of animal used, septic insult chosen and time of evolution [31, 32].

The increase in renal blood flow is in a global manner and there is no difference between the cortical and medullar layer. Observations carried out through analysis of flow by Doppler fluxometry showed normal flow between the cortical and medullar layer in patients with sepsis.

However, there is need for more studies and the technology used for this analysis is a crucial factor for the intra-renal flow specification [33]. Septic patients are often resuscitated with huge amounts of fluid infusion besides the infusion of antimicrobial drugs and vasoactive agents which results in a positive fluid balance day after day. This volume overload leads to an increase in glomerular blood pressure and reduced renal perfusion which contributes to the AKI development [34].

Nonhemodynamic Factors

Thenon-hemodynamic factors of significance are the release of inflammatory mediators such as tumor necrosis factor-alpha, interleukins, metabolites of arachidonic acid, vasoactive substances and two mechanisms of cell death, necrosis and apoptosis. Discussing the whole inflammatory pathway with its facilitators and inhibitors is beyond the objective of this chapter [31].

Table 3. Dialysis Methods—this table is associated with the text on page 12

	IHD	SLED	SCUF	CVVH	CVVHD	CVVHDF	PD
Blood Flow Rate ml/min	250-400	100-200	<100	200-300	100-200	100-200	
Dyalisate Flow ml/min	500-800	100	0	0	16.7-33.4	16.7-33.4	0.4
Filtrate L/day	0-4	0-4	0-4	24-96	0	24-48	2.4
Replacement Fluid L/day	0	0	0	21.6-90	4.8	23-44	0
Solute Clearence Mechanism	Diffusion	Diffusion	Convection	Convection	Diffusion	Both	Both
Duration(h)	3-4	8-12	Variable	>24	>24	>24	

Adapted from Mehta RL. Continuous renal replacement therapy in the critically ill patient. Kidney Int. 2005;67:781-95.

Abbreviations: IHD: intermittent hemodialysis, SCUF:slow- continuous hemofiltration; CVVH: continuous venofiltration hemofiltration; CVVHD: continuous venovenous hemodialysis; CVVHDF: continuous venovenous hemodiafiltration.

TNF Alpha

The TNF alpha is an important mediator in sepsis induced by Gram-negative bacteria. It is released in kidneys by mesangial cells after stimulation by lipopolysaccharide (LPS). Systemically, during the septic insult, it promotes tissue hypo perfusion, apoptosis, and fibrin deposition and stimulates the migration of leukocytes. Despite its functional role as inflammatory mediator, only recently, through the development of techniques of its blockade, it has been observed experimentally that TNF alpha could exert a protective effect on the glomerular filtration rate in a sepsis model using rats treated and not treated with a blocker of its action [33].

Cunningham et al. showed that mice deficient in TNF receptors had greater resistance to renal injury induced by sepsis following infusion of LPS [35]. These observations suggest an important immunological role in the genesis of acute kidney injury in patients with sepsis.

Interleukin -6

The IL 6 is an important mediator of fever and acute phase of the inflammatory response. It is produced and secreted by T lymphocytes and macrophages. Its action in sepsis is well known and its increasing levels being directly related to the prognosis and evolution of sepsis. [36] Chawla et al. pointed out that the higher the level of IL 6, the greater the APACHE prognostic score is. Therefore there is a higher chance for the patient with sepsis and high levels of IL6to develop acute kidney injury [37].

A recent clinical study correlated the levels of some mediators of acute phase reaction in patients with sepsis, among them the interleukin 6, and the degree of severity of kidney injury as well as the necessity for dialysis and mortality. It was observed that patients who developed severe acute kidney injury, defined by present classification AKIN 3, had higher mortality and higher levels of interleukin 6 compared with the other groups with kidney injury [38].

Necrosis and Apoptosis

The entire insult generated by sepsis at cellular level may trigger the process of death by two ways: necrosis or apoptosis.

The cellular necrosis occurs when the cell is depleted of energy, ATP, and evolves to the collapse of its homeostasis in an uncoordinated manner. The apoptosis, programmed death, occurs in an active manner that is with energy expenditure, is chemically activated and is characterized by chromatin condensation, nuclear rupture, vacuolization of the plasma membrane and cell shrinkage. Levine, in 2001, first reported that apoptosis could be a mechanism of acute kidney injury in sepsis. Periods of ischemia are responsible for triggering of apoptotic bodies around 24 hours after the initial insult. The period of ischemia can vary but within 5 minutes of injury it is possible to observe the mechanism described above [39].

Measures to prevent apoptosis include the administration of mediators which can block the biochemical signaling by specific receptors for the cell death programming. Among them are the inhibitors of caspase, an enzyme which is believed to have a crucial role in intra-cellular signaling for the initiation of apoptosis [39].

Treatment

In general, the treatment of AKI in sepsis is supportive care, maintenance of normal glucose levels, early antimicrobial therapy, appropriate attention to the site of infection, adequate mechanical ventilation. Diuretics usage is beneficial in the treatment of AKI only in hypervolemia states and should not delay the initiation of dialysis when indicated. Even with a good urine output, the pharmacologic intervention to withdraw fluid is ineffective as monotherapy.

Dialysis Modalities

The choice of dialysis method must fit what the patient needs. Table 3 presents the advantages and disadvantages of each dialysis method. The results of the studies are conflicting as a consequence of multiple comorbidities common to these patients, heterogeneity in the definition of early initiation of dialysis and the improvement in outcome at 30 days for example is only due to this variable (start time).

There is the possibility of performing SLED instead of continuous therapy (CVVHD) with good results for the clearance of medium molecules and urea. However, the intermittent dialysis (IHD) offers more risk of hemodynamic complications during its implementation.

Continuous methods are associated with less hemodynamic instability in part because of a less fluid withdraw per hour. However as a continuous method it allows a higher withdraw in 24 hours than extended or intermittent methods.

References

[1] Angus DC, Linde-Zwirble WT, Lidicker J, Clermont G, Carcillo J, Pinsky MR. Epidemiology of severe sepsis in the United States: analysis of incidence, outcome, and associated costs of care. *Crit. Care Med.* 2001 Jul;29(7):1303-10.

[2] Hall MJ, Williams SN, De Frances CJ, Golosinskiy A. Inpatient care for septicemia or sepsis: A challenge for patients and hospitals. NCHS data brief, no 62. Hyattsville, MD: *National Center for Health Statistics*. 2011.

[3] Case J, Khan S, Khalid R, Khan A. Epidemiology of acute kidney injury in the intensive care unit. *Crit. Care. Res. Pract.* 2013;2013:479730. doi: 10.1155 /2013 /479730.

[4] Chertow GM, Burdick E, Honour M, Bonventre JV, Bates DW. Acute kidney injury, mortality, length of stay, and costs in hospitalized patients. *J. Am. Soc. Nephrol.* 2005 Nov;16(11):3365-70.

[5] Wang HE, Muntner P, Chertow GM, Warnock DG. Acute kidney injury and mortality in hospitalized patients. *Am. J. Nephrol.* 2012;35(4):349-55. doi: 10.1159/000337487.

[6] Bagshaw SM, Lapinsky S, Dial S, Arabi Y, Dodek P, Wood G, Ellis P, Guzman J, Marshall J, Parrillo JE, Skrobik Y, Kumar A; Cooperative Antimicrobial Therapy of Septic Shock (CATSS) Database Research Group. Acute kidney injury in septic shock: clinical outcomes and impact of duration of hypotension prior to initiation of

antimicrobial therapy. *Intensive Care. Med.* 2009 May;35(5):871-81. doi: 10.1007 /s00134-008-1367-2.

[7] Levy MM, Fink MP, Marshall JC, Abraham E, Angus D, Cook D, Cohen J, Opal SM, Vincent JL, Ramsay G; SCCM/ESICM/ACCP/ATS/SIS. 2001 SCCM/ESICM/ ACCP/ATS/SIS International Sepsis Definitions Conference. *Crit. Care. Med.* 2003 Apr;31(4):1250-6.

[8] Dellinger RP, Levy MM, Rhodes A, Annane D, Gerlach H, Opal SM, Sevransky JE, Sprung CL, Douglas IS, Jaeschke R, Osborn TM, Nunnally ME, Townsend SR, Reinhart K, Kleinpell RM, Angus DC, Deutschman CS, Machado FR, Rubenfeld GD, Webb SA, Beale RJ, Vincent JL, Moreno R; Surviving Sepsis Campaign Guidelines Committee including the Pediatric Subgroup. Surviving sepsis campaign: international guidelines for management of severe sepsis and septic shock: 2012. *Crit. Care. Med.* 2013 Feb;41(2):580-637.doi:10.1097/CCM.0b013e31827e83af.

[9] Sharfudin A, Weisbord SD, Pavlesky PM, Molitoris BA. Acute Kidney Injury. In: Brenner& Rector´s The Kidney 9th edition edited by Taal MW et al. Elsevier 2012: pp1044-1099.

[10] Bellomo R, Ronco C, Kellum JA, et al. Acute renal failure - definition, outcome measures, animal models, fluid therapy and information technology needs: the Second International Consensus Conference of the Acute Dialysis Quality Initiative (ADQI) Group. *Crit. Care.* 2004; 8: R204–212.

[11] Kidney Disease: Improving Global Outcomes (KDIGO) Acute Kidney Injury Work Group. KDIGO Clinical Practice Guideline for Acute Kidney Injury. *Kidney inter., Suppl.* 2012; 2: 1–138.

[12] Levey AS, Bosch JP, Lewis JB, Greene T, Rogers N, Roth D: A more accurate method to estimate glomerular filtration rate from serum creatinine: a new prediction equation. Modification of Diet in Renal Disease Study Group. *Ann. Intern. Med.* 1999; 130: 461–470.

[13] Levey AS, Stevens LA, Schmid CH, Zhang YL, Castro AF, Feldman HI et al. A new equation to estimate glomerular filtration rate. *Ann. Intern. Med.* 2009 May 5; 150(9): 604-12.

[14] Bragadottir G, Redfors B, Ricksten SE. Assessing glomerular filtration rate (GFR) in critically ill patients with acute kidney injury - true GFR versus urinary creatinine clearance and estimating equations. *Crit. Care.* 2013 Jun 15;17(3):R108.

[15] Chen S. Retooling the creatinine clearance equation to estimate kinetic GFR when the plasma creatinine is changing acutely.*J. Am. Soc. Nephrol.* 2013 May;24(6):877-88. doi: 10.1681/ASN.2012070653. Epub 2013 May 23.

[16] Macedo E, Bouchard J, Soroko SH, Chertow GM, Himmelfarb J, Ikizler TA, Paganini EP, Mehta RL. Program to Improve Care in Acute Renal Disease Study. Fluid accumulation, recognition and staging of acute kidney injury in critically-ill patients. *Crit. Care.* 2010;14(3):R82. doi: 10.1186/cc9004.

[17] Cerda J, Cerda M, Kilcullen P, Prendergast J. In severe acute kidney injury, a higher serum creatinine is paradoxically associated with better patient survival. *Nephrol. Dial. Transplant.* 2007 Oct;22.

[18] Haase-Fielitz A, Bellomo R, Devarajan P, Story D, Matalanis G, Dragun D, Haase M. Novel and conventional sérum biomarkers predicting acute kidney injury in adult cardiac surgery- a prospective cohort study. *Crit. Care. Med.* 2009;37:553-60.

[19] McIlroy DR, Wagener G, Lee HT. Biomarkers of acute kidney injury: an evolving domain. *Anesthesiology* 2010 Apr;112(4):998-1004. doi: 10.1097 /ALN. 0b013e3181cded3f.

[20] Shlipak MG, Matsushita K, Ärnlöv J, Inker LA, Katz R, Polkinghorne KR, Rothenbacher D, Sarnak MJ, Astor BC, Coresh J, Levey AS, Gansevoort RT; CKD Prognosis Consortium. Cystatin C versus Creatinine in Determining Risk Based on Kidney Function. *N. Engl. J. Med.* 2013 Sep 5;369(10):932-43. doi: 10.1056 /NEJMoa1214234.

[21] Endre ZH, Goldstein SL, Somma S, Doi K, Macedo E, Kellum JA, Mehta RL. Differential Diagnosis of AKI in Clinical Practice by Functional and Damage Biomarkers: Workgroup Statements from the Tenth Acute Dialysis Quality Initiative Consensus Conference. *Contributions to Nephrology* 2013;182:30-44.

[22] Mishra J, dent C, Tarabishi R, Mitsnefes MM, Ma Q, Kelly C, Ruff SM, Zahedi K, Shao M , Bean J et al. Neutrophil gelatinase-associated lipocalin(NGAL) as a biomarker for acute renal injury after cardiac surgery. *Lancet.* 2005;365:1231-8.

[23] Metra M, Cotter G, Gheorghiade M, Dei Cas L, Voors AA. The role of the kidney in heart failure. *Eur. Heart J.* 2012 Sep;33(17):2135-42. doi: 10.1093/eurheartj/ehs205.

[24] Haase M, Bellomo R, Devarajan P, Schlattmann P, Haase-Fielitz A; NGAL Meta-analysis Investigator Group. Accuracy of neutrophil gelatinase-associated lipocalin (NGAL) in diagnosis and prognosis in acute kidney injury: a systematic review and meta-analysis. *Am. J. Kidney Dis.* 2009 Dec;54(6):1012-24. doi: 10.1053/j.ajkd. 2009.07.020.

[25] Glassford NJ, Schneider AG, Xu S, Eastwood GM, Young H, Peck L, Venge P, Bellomo R. The nature and discriminatory value of urinary neutrophil gelatinase-associated lipocalin in critically ill patients at risk of acute kidney injury. *Intensive Care Med.* 2013;39:1714-24.

[26] Doi K, Yuen PS, Eisner C, Hu X, Leelahavanichkul A, Schnermann J, Star RA. Reduced production of creatinine limits its use as marker of kidney injury in sepsis. *J. Am. Soc. Nephrol.* 2009:20: 1217-21.

[27] Nejat M, Hill JV, Pickering JW, Edelstein CL, Devarajan P, Endre ZH: Albuminuria increases cystatin C excretion: implications for urinary biomarkers. *Nephrol. Dial. Transpl.* 2011.

[28] Langenberg C, Bagshaw SM, May CN, Bellomo R.The histopathology of septic acute kidney injury: a systematic review. *Crit. Care.* 2008;12(2):R38. doi: 10.1186/cc6823.

[29] Ravikant T, Lucas CE. Renal blood flow distribution in septic hyperdynamic pigs. *J. Surg. Res.* 1977 Mar;22(3):294-8.

[30] Brenner M, Schaer GL, Mallory DL, Suffredini AF, Parrillo JE. Detection of renal blood flow abnormalities in septic and critically ill patients using a newly designed indwelling thermodilution renal vein catheter. *Chest.* 1990 Jul;98(1):170-9.

[31] Wan L, Bellomo R, Di Giantomasso D, Ronco C. The pathogenesis of septic acute renal failure. *Curr. Opin. Crit. Care.* 2003 Dec;9(6):496-502.

[32] Zarjou A, Agarwal A. Sepsis and acute kidney injury.. *J. Am. Soc. Nephrol.* 2011 Jun;22(6):999-1006. doi: 10.1681/ASN.2010050484.

[33] Knotek M, Rogachev B, Wang W, Ecder T, Melnikov V, Gengaro PE, Esson M, Edelstein CL, Dinarello CA, Schrier RW. Endotoxemic renal failure in mice: Role of

tumor necrosis factor independent of inducible nitric oxide synthase. *Kidney Int*. 2001 Jun;59(6):2243-9.

[34] Cerda J.Oliguria: an earlier and accurate biomarker of acute kidney injury? *Kidney Int*. 2011 Oct;80(7):699-701. doi: 10.1038/ki.2011.177.

[35] Cunningham PN, Dyanov HM, Park P, Wang J, Newell KA, Quigg RJ. Acute renal failure in endotoxemia is caused by TNF acting directly on TNF receptor-1 in kidney. *J. Immunol*. 2002 Jun 1;168(11):5817-23.

[36] Marshall JC, Vincent JL, Fink MP, Cook DJ, Rubenfeld G, Foster D, Fisher CJ Jr, Faist E, Reinhart K. Measures, markers, and mediators: toward a staging system for clinical sepsis. A report of the Fifth Toronto Sepsis Roundtable, Toronto, Ontario, Canada, October 25-26, 2000. *Crit. Care. Med*. 2003 May;31(5):1560-7.

[37] Chawla LS, Seneff MG, Nelson DR, Williams M, Levy H, Kimmel PL, Macias WL. Elevated plasma concentrations of IL-6 and elevated APACHE II score predict acute kidney injury in patients with severe sepsis. *Clin. J. Am. Soc. Nephrol*. 2007 Jan;2(1):22-30.

[38] Payen D, Lukaszewicz AC, Legrand M, Gayat E, Faivre V, Megarbane B, Azoulay E, Fieux F, Charron D, Loiseau P, Busson M. A multicentre study of acute kidney injury in severe sepsis and septic shock: association with inflammatory phenotype and HLA genotype. *PLoS One*. 2012;7(6):e35838. doi: 10.1371/journal.pone.0035838.

[39] Levine JS, Lieberthal W: Terminal pathways to cell death. *In Acute Renal*.

[40] Failure First edition. Edited by Molitoris BA, Finn WF. New York: WB Saunders; 2001:30–59.21.

[41] Mehta RL. Continuous renal replacement therapy in the critically ill patient. *Kidney Int*. 2005;67:781-95.

In: Sepsis
Editor: Nancy Khardori

ISBN: 978-1-63117-244-1

Chapter 4

Prevention of Hospital-Acquired Infection with Focus on Sepsis in Neonatal Intensive Care Units: Use of Quality Improvement Efforts

Adolf Valls-i-Soler, M.D., Ph.D.[1,2], *Marisela Madrid*[2] *BSB., Agueda Azpeitia*[2] *and Elena Santesteban*[2] *Ph.D.*

[1]Neonatal Intensive

[2]Neonatal Epidemiology Units, Cruces University Hospital, University of the Basque country, Bilbao, Spain

Abstract

In neonates, HAI is usually defined as presence of clinical signs of systemic infection with or without a positive blood culture, appearing after the first 72 hours of life. Premature infants are more susceptible to infections due to added immaturity of the immune system. They remain in a critical state for weeks, require prolonged and complex care provided by numerous caregivers, and are in need for invasive life-support techniques (intravascular catheters, intubation and mechanical ventilation). Furthermore, late-onset sepsis is a major cause of mortality and morbidity in preterm infants who suffer from complications like intraventricular haemorrhage, bronchopulmonary dysplasia, necrotizing enterocholitis... with a 2.5-fold increase in mortality and more than 30% increase in the length of hospital stay in culture-proven sepsis.

In Europe, data from *EuroNeoStat* project shows that between 2006-2011, the HAI prevalence in over 190 European neonatal intensive care units was 25.2% (95%CI: 24.7-25.7%). Despite advances in neonatal intensive care and antimicrobials, mortality rate was higher in babies with late-onset sepsis (15.2 vs. 12.9%), OR=1.21 (95%CI: 1.1-1.3). HAI increases the likelihood of an adverse neurodevelopmental outcome, including cerebral palsy, low mental and psychomotor development index, and vision impairment.

It is well recognized that HAI is potentially preventable, the estimated preventable proportion being between 10 and 70%, depending on the setting, baseline infection rates and type of infection. Nowadays, HAI prevention in hospital settings involves benchmarking and the implementation of surveillance systems and safe clinical practices. Several neonatal networks have done just that; providing valuable information for benchmarking between units and allowing the design of intervention strategies and public health policies that improve the quality of care of these high-risk patients.

Models currently used for prevention of infection are evidence-based, and combine interventions built-in continuous quality improvement initiatives. These models exemplify the integration of results of clinical research into daily clinical practice; aiming to provide high quality care, focused on systems that tend to be error-free in the implementation of effective change and to assess its impact. These combined interventions are based on the recollection and diffusion of scientific evidence and the simultaneous application of a set of preventive measures along with the establishment of an environment of intense multidisciplinary collaboration, to design and develop plans to improve the quality of care.

To establish a successful program to prevent HAI, the use of the Plan-Do-Study-Act-cycle multiple bundle methodology is strongly recommended, as it has been shown effective. It must also be based on evidence, team learning and acting, and above all on a culture for patient safety.

Abbreviations

CDC	Centers for Disease Control and Prevention
CNN	Canadian Neonatal Network
EuroNeoNet	European Neonatal Network
HAI	Hospital-acquired infection
KISS	Krankenhaus-Infektions-Surveillance-System
NEO-KISS	Krankenhaus-Infektions-Surveillance-System for neonates
NNIS	National Nosocomial Infection Surveillance
NICUs	Neonatal Intensive Care Units
SIRS	systemic inflammation response syndrome
VLBW	Very Low Birth Weight
VLGA	Very Low Gestational Age
WHO	World Health Organization

Introduction

The aim of this chapter is to outline the prevalence and immediate and long term adverse consequences of Hospital-acquired infection (HAI) in newborn infants. More specifically, the importance of its prevention, a possible but not an easy task, will be reviewed.

After completing this chapter, readers should be able to:

1. Describe the epidemiology of HAI in Very Low Birth Weight (VLBW) infants and its short and long term consequences.
2. Explain the importance of surveillance for HAI in preterm infants.
3. Describe strategies and processes that may help to decrease the rate of HAI in Neonatal Intensive Care Units (NICUs).

Infection still is a global health problem affecting neonates, infants and children around the world. The World Health Organization (WHO) has emphasized the important contribution of infection to neonatal mortality, since of the 5 million neonatal deaths per year worldwide, a quarter are related to neonatal sepsis and/or pneumonia.

Case fatality rates for neonatal infections in developing countries remain much higher for hospitalized newborns [1] and for those cared for in the community. [2,3] Infection is mainly related to unsafe birth practices, and thus its prevention must be centred on achieving sterile conditions during birth and umbilical cord care.

On the other hand, in developed countries bacterial infections occurring in the first three days of life might result from intrapartum exposure to maternal genital microorganisms. However, an increasing percentage of neonatal infections have their onset beyond this age, and are in fact caused by nosocomial pathogens. [4] Thus, severe bloodstream infection affects almost exclusively newborn infants in need of life support techniques in NICUs, mainly prematurely born infants but some with other conditions like congenital malformations.

HAI might complicate the hospital course of any sick newborn infant requiring intensive care, but its prevalence increases as gestational age decreases. HAI affects one out of 50 term newborn infants admitted to NICUs [5,6]. However, its prevalence in premature babies of very low gestational age (VLGA) and/or very low birth weight (VLBW) is much higher, one out of 4 of such infants. [6,7]

To fully understand the great impact of HAI in VLGA infants, it should be noted that every year over 15 million babies are born prematurely worldwide, about 16% (2,400,000) of them before 32 weeks of gestation. Premature birth is in theory preventable, but its prevalence is rising in developed and developing countries. The 2012 WHO´s report *"Born Too Soon. Global Action Report on Premature Birth"* showed prematurity to be among the greatest health hazards of humankind and the single most common cause of mortality, morbidity and disability, being the second cause of child mortality after pneumonia, overtaking diarrhea and malaria, and responsible for 1.1 million deaths a year. [8]

Hospital-Acquired Infections in Neonates

VLGA/VLBW infants are at highest risk for HAI, since they remain in acute care for extended periods, and require complex life-support techniques (e.g. intubation, mechanical ventilation, intravascular catheters for parental nutrition) provided by numerous care givers. In VLBW infants, HAI is responsible for a 2.5-fold increase in neonatal mortality and the rates of all major neonatal morbidities (intraventricular hemorrhage, periventricular leukomalatia, chronic lung disease) [9], and increase in the length of hospital stays [7]. In turn, these conditions further increase the need for invasive life-support interventions which further prolongs the length of hospital stay and thus the risk for HAI.

To precisely illustrate the real impact of HAI in immature infants of VLGA, data from EuroNeoNet (European Neonatal Network funded since 2006 by the European Commission's DGSANCO; www.euroneonet.org) is provided. Between 2006 and 2011 the overall prevalence of HAI in over 190 European NICUs was 25.2% (95% Confidence Interval (CI):24.7-25.7%) with a wide inter-centre variability (1.8 to 63.1%) (Figure 1).

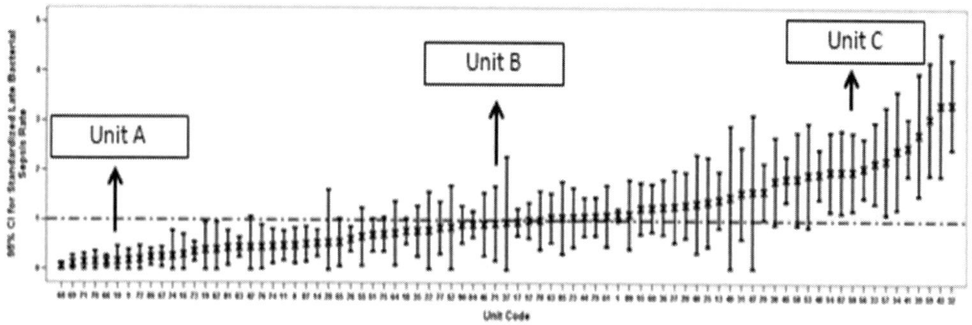

Figure 1. Standardized rate of Late Onset Sepsis (LOS). (EuroNeoNet 2011 Report). This rate and its 95% CI are calculated to provide relative risk estimation between the standard global population and that of each NICU. Reference rates are applied to the populations compared, standardizing by confounding factors. This result is the expected number of cases of LOS for each NICU. If the observed number of LOS cases is divided by the expected number, the standardised LOS rate is obtained. Thus, if the 95%CI is completely below (unit A) or above (unit C) the 1 line, the LOS rate for those specific NICUs are significantly below or above the standardized LOS rate. Otherwise the LOS rate is average (Unit B).

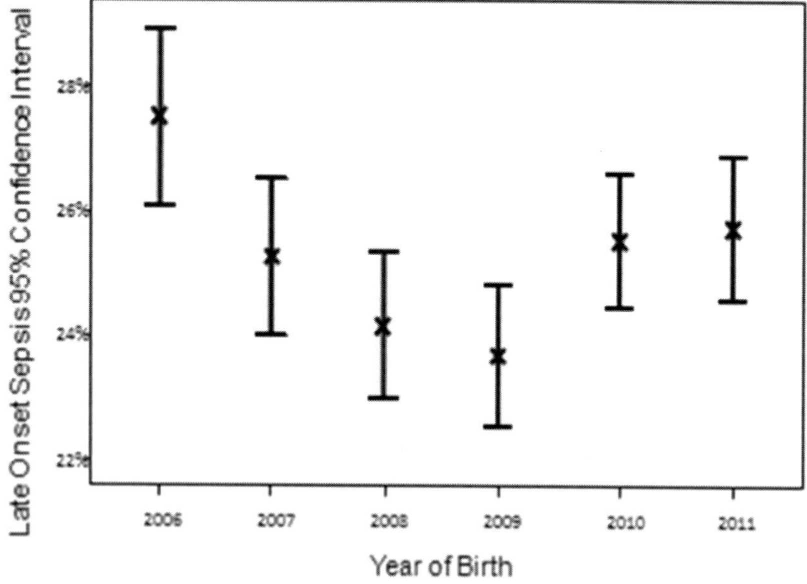

Figure 2. Late Onset Sepsis Rates and its 95% Confidence Interval by year of birth. Population excludes deaths in delivery room and babies with a gestational age above 32. (EuroNeoNet 2011 Report).

Despite this inter-center variability, the annual rates of HAI have remained stable in the six years studied, ranging from 23 to 27% (Figure 2).VLBW infants who developed HAI had a higher neonatal mortality rate (15.2 vs. 12.9%; Odd Ratio (OR):1.21 (95% CI: 1.1-1.3). Moreover, they were also at greater risk for severe morbidities such as bronchopulmonary dysplasia (35.2 vs. 13.7%; OR:3.4; 95% CI:3.15-3.73); necrotizing enterocolitis (14.7 vs. 3.8%; OR:4.3; 95%CI:3.96-4.76); severe intraventricular hemorrhage (12.2 vs. 8.2%; OR:1.6;

95%CI:1.43-1.69); periventricular leukomalacia (8.8 vs. 4.8%; OR:1.9; 95%CI:1.72-2.1) and severe retinopathy of prematurity (9.6 vs.3.0%; OR:3.4; 95%CI:3-3.88).In Spain, data from the "Grupo Castrillo" registry [6] of neonatal infections from 35 NICUs, show that in 2011 the incidence of HAI was 29.9% (3,404 episodes of bloodstream infections in 11,357 VLBW infants), being the incidence density of 5.9 episodes by 1.000 days of hospital stay. [6] Like in EuroNeoNet, in the Spanish registry the overall rate of HAI remained stable over the same six year period.

Long-Term Consequences of HAI

It should be stressed that decreasing HAI not only means saving lives but also increasing the number of handicap-free years. The impact of avoiding one case of a neonate with severe handicap on the society is very large, because the life expectancy of a neonate is much longer compared to an adult patient suffering from a similar disease. Therefore, the overall effects of avoiding handicapped children from the neonatal population on the emotional burden for the families and the economic impact on the society is tremendous.

HAI increases the likelihood of an adverse neurodevelopmental outcome, including cerebral palsy (ORs range 1.4-1.7), low mental (ORs: 1.3-1.6) and psychomotor development index (ORs: 1.5-2.4), and vision impairment (ORs: 1.3-2.2). [10] In addition, educational, behavioural and social impairments are prevalent among HAI survivors. [11]

The consequences of prematurity pose major financial costs on families, health care systems and society. Neonatal infection has been estimated to double the costs of care of VLBW from US$ 6,200 to 12.480 [12, 13]. EuroNeoNet data also shows the burden of HAI increases health care costs, since it increases the length of hospital stay of babies discharged home (78.7±37.7 vs. 54.2±26.2 days). Moreover, the life-long economic costs of a patient with cerebral palsy have been estimated to be about €800.000. Other studies also have quantified the costs of mental retardation, hearing and vision impairment, all known to be associated with infection and its therapy. [14]

It should be considered that the long term consequences of HAI go far beyond all those economic impacts, producing continued stress to parents, families. Furthermore, care-givers do feel somehow responsible for it, and thus are especially motivated to undertake preventive actions.

Prevention of HAI in Intensive Care Units

Of the many steps required to successfully decrease the rate of HAI in neonates, the first one is to implement an effective and sustainable monitoring system specifically designed for neonatal intensive care areas. Most importantly, a standardized definition must be used to measure the infectious events, allowing NICU to objectively measure the magnitude of the problem and evaluate the effects of the preventive measures that have been implemented. Furthermore, the plan should also permit comparisons of rates with other NICUs of similar case load and case mix.

Definition of Neonatal Septic Episodes

For neonatal infections, classification according to transmission mechanism -vertical or perinatal and postnatal or horizontal- is used, since etiological organisms and morbidity and mortality rates are different. However, sometimes it is difficult to clearly establish this distinction.

Neonatal networks developed the concepts of early and late onset sepsis if the symptoms start before or after the first 3 days of life respectively. Assuming this scheme, early onset sepsis is always assumed to be of perinatal transmission, and late onset sepsis of horizontal transmission, also known as HAI. [15] However, this chronological classification can also be misleading, since although most septic episodes due to vertical transmission start in the first 3 days of life, they may initiate beyond the third day. Similarly, noscomial or HAI may present in the first three days of life.

In neonates, sepsis is difficult to diagnose and no consensus exists about its definition among clinicians and researchers. In fact, different definitions are used to select patients to receive early optimal therapy, to enroll them in clinical trials or for surveillance propose. [16] To select neonates for early treatment, the concepts of "suspected" or "probable" and "possible" sepsis are used. However, in VLGA infants, in whom sepsis is more frequent and treated, between 25 and 50% receive antibiotics for clinically diagnosed septic episodes that are later found culture-negative. [17,18,19] This is related among other reasons, to frequent use of antibiotic in the mother, insufficient blood volume obtained problems which are even more evident in VLBW infants.

In order to include newborn infants in clinical trials to evaluate the safety and efficacy of antimicrobials, an operational definition has been proposed, to stimulate the development of such drugs since none of them have been evaluated thoroughly in this population. [20]

Definition of neonatal HAI Episodes for Surveillance

Finally, for surveillance of HAI in acute care hospital settings, the Centers for Disease Control and Prevention (CDC) defined sepsis as a localized or systemic condition resulting from an adverse reaction to the presence of an infectious agent(s) or its toxin(s), with no evidence that it was present or incubating at the time of admission. [21] Later, systemic inflammation response syndrome (SIRS) with fever, increased heart, respiratory rate and white cell count was defined to which evidence of organ dysfunction was added. [22] However, this definition is not useful for children, much less for newborn infants; who frequently do not manifest the typical early signs of SIRS or multiple organ failure, since their response to infection is frequently delayed, attenuated or nonexistent, like in VLBW infants with late onset sepsis.

For monitoring neonatal HAI in VLGA infants, several definitions have been suggested. For benchmarking proposes, neonatal networks have developed an operational definition used by most of them (Table 1). [15]

Late onset sepsis is used as a surrogate for HAI, defined as infection after 3 days (or 72 hours) of life with a positive blood and/or cerebral spinal fluid culture for pathogenic organisms (EuroNeoNet).

Table 1. Definitions of Hospital-acquired infection by a neonatal network and neonatal surveillance system

European Neonatal Network (EuroNeoNet), Spain (2006) http://www.euroneonet.eu/paginas/publicas/euroneo/euroNeoNet/ennet_documents.htm.
Late sepsis and/or meningitis (after 72 hours of birth) a) *Laboratory-confirmed bloodstream infection. (except Staphylococcus epidermidis).* Patient has a pathogen recovered from a blood and/or cerebrospinal fluid culture obtained after day 3 of life. *b) Laboratory-confirmed bloodstream infection with Coagulase-negative Staphylococci* Patient must meet *ALL* of the following conditions: Coagulase-negative Stapylococci is recovered from a blood culture obtained from either a central line, or peripheral blood simple and/or is recovered from cerebrospinal fluid obtained by lumbar puncture, ventricular tap or ventricular drain. Signs of generalized infection (such as apnea, temperature instability, feeding intolerance, worsening respiratory distress or hemodynamic instability). Treatment with 5 or more days of intravenous antibiotics after the above cultures was obtained. If the infant died, was discharged, or transferred prior to the completion of 5 days of intravenous antibiotics, this condition would still be met if the intention were to treat for 5 or more days.
Krankenhaus Infections Surveillance System for preterm infants (Neo-Kiss) Germany (2000) [15] http://www.nrz-hygiene.de/en/surveillance/hospital-infection-surveillance-system/neo-kiss/
Two the following clinical criteria must be met in all forms of bloodstream infection *At least two of:* temperature >38.0°C or <36.5°C or temperature instability, tachycardia or bradycardia, apnea, prolonged capillary refill, metabolic acidosis, hyperglycemia, other signs of bloodstream infection such as decreased responsiveness. *In addition to the clinical criteria the following condition must meet:* *Criteria for Clinically Suspected Bloodstream Infection: (infection without a detected pathogen) AND* • Blood cultures not performed or results of blood cultures or antigen tests in blood are negative.
• No apparent infection at another site. • Physician prescribes antibiotic treatment for bloodstream infection. *Criteria for Laboratory-confirmed Bloodstream Infection (Not coagulase negative Staphylococci) AND* • A recognized pathogen other than coagulase-negative staphylococci cultured from blood or cerebrospinal fluid. • The organism is not related to an infection at another site. *Criteria for Laboratory-confirmed Bloodstream Infection with coagulase-negative Staphylococci. AND* • Coagulase-negative Staphylococci is cultured from blood. Patient has one of: C-reactive protein >2.0 mg/dl or increased interleukin 6 through 8, immature/total neutrophil ratio (I/T-ratio) >0.2, leukocytes $<5.0x10^3/\mu l$ (<5/nl), platelets$<100x10^3/\mu l$ (<100/nl)

The number of infants with infection per 100 infants admitted is used as an indicator for comparison. However, this definition has several drawbacks related to lack of inclusion of frequent culture-negative clinical sepsis, no accounting of repetitive septic episodes, and especially that although standardized for gestational age or other risk factors, is not directly related to key factors like use and length of indwelling catheters and duration of stay. *Staphylococcus epidermidis,* once thought benign and non pathogenic, is now recognized as the most frequent organism causing HAI in VLGA infants. [7] However, since contamination can occur at the time of blood sampling or during processing, because of its ubiquitous presence on the skin of health care and laboratory workers, it remains possible that some of these episodes might represent a contamination. To solve this problem, two successive positive blood cultures from peripheral blood specimens are required for diagnosis.

Monitoring Systems for Bloodstream Infections

Great efforts have been put into the surveillance and prevention of HAI, now recognised as an important problem of patient safety, affecting quality of care, being responsible for significant morbidity and mortality, especially in patients admitted to intensive care units. [5,23,24,25]

Due to their severe nature and adverse short and long term consequences, neonatal infection surveillance in NICUs is usually limited to bloodstream bacterial infections and fungi like *candida* species. Unlike in adult and pediatric intensive care areas, where infections are monitored in all patients admitted, in neonates surveillance can be limited to VLGA/VLBW infants. This high risk population is ideal for monitoring and assessing the impact of any preventive measures being implemented. The assumption is that if HAI decreases in this population, same will happen in the rest of the neonatal population in need of intensive care, since measures necessary to prevent infections depend mainly on the type of medical procedures.

Nowadays, the state-of-the-art in HAI monitoring in hospital settings basically involves benchmarking by neonatal networks for quality assurance ,achieving a standardized rate similar to that of other units, the implementation of specific surveillance systems specially designed and validated for their use in newborn infants and the implementation of safe and evidence-based clinical practices for quality improvement with the goal of achieving a rate similar to units with the lowest rates. Common to both quality assessment methods is the need to use harmonized definitions and standardized indicators for surveillance of HAI.

Benchmarking of HAI by Neonatal Networks

Networking has been used to improve the quality of health care by disseminating information on evidence-based effective and ineffective or dangerous interventions (e.g., by the Cochrane Collaboration) and promoting high quality research. Neonatal networking can be defined as a collaborative work involving several NICUs sharing a common protocol aimed to collect standardized patient data for external audits (benchmarking), clinical trials, and quality of care improvement projects. [26]

Neonatal networks have a long standing record of performing quality assessment of several adverse outcomes, like infection, to allow individual NICUs to assure that the observed rate of adverse event or outcome is not outside a standardized range achieved by other NICUs of the network.

The National Nosocomial Infection Surveillance (NNIS) Report developed by the CDC, [21] has been used as a standard for monitoring infection in neonates. Networks not only provide valuable information to participating NICUs for benchmarking, but also help in designing and evaluating different intervention to improve the quality of care of neonates, specifically by infection prevention. [26,27]

> Comparisons using network data is based on risk adjustments for perinatal and neonatal risk factors and outcome measures. However, heterogeneity present after those adjustments might be attributable to factors other than quality of care, such as case mix, quality of data, babies´ length of stay and invasive medical procedures, all of which can influence HAI. [28] To make fair and meaningful comparisons between hospitals, a multicentre monitoring system must also adjust for these factors, using not only outcome but process indicators, usually related to number of catheter days and length of stay as denominators. [5] Accordingly, surveillance systems developed for use in neonates, centered on risk for VLGA infants, use infection density standardized indicators per 100 days of catheter´ use or 1000 patient days in the NICU. [23]

Surveillance of Neonatal HAI by Specific Monitoring System

In pediatric and adult intensive care areas, HAI monitoring is performed in all patients, since all are considered at risk. In NICUs, large numbers of patients are assisted but have heterogeneous characteristics and risks, requiring clearly different levels of care intensity. Thus, only those babies at highest risk for HAI, precisely infants of VLGA/VLBW during their initial critical period, are usually screened. It is assumed that an improvement in this population will be accompanied by a decrease in HAI patients at lower risk and/or more mature.

The implementation of standardized, well evaluated surveillance systems for HAI in newborn infants has been rather scarce. In Europe, to provide hospitals with standard surveillance methods some projects and national infection surveillance systems were developed for adults and paediatric population in the nineties. [29]

In Germany, from the "Krankenhaus-Infektions-Surveillance-System (KISS)" a specific component for VLBW infants (Neo-Kiss) was developed by an expert panel of neonatologists and tested in a pilot project. [23,29] Neo-Kiss is mainly focussed on surveillance of bloodstream infection, pneumonia and necrotizing enterocholitis and studies their correlation to catheters, ventilator devices and the use of antibiotics. At present, a total of 220 German neonatal centres are participating in this highly successful networking effort. [30]

Neo-Kiss modified the original CDC definition adjusting it to the specific characteristics of VLBW infants. Because of the high level of agreement between the CDC and the modified criteria for the central line-associated blood stream infection and ventilator-associated pneumonia, they decided to use the modified definitions that nonetheless would allow comparisons with NNIS data. [31] Neo-Kiss data suggest that participation in ongoing surveillance of HAI with feedback data to individual units, may lead to a reduction of HAI in

VLBW infants. The incidence density of HAI decreased significantly by 24% (from 8.3 per 1000 patient-days in the first year to 6.4 in the third year of its implementation; OR 0.73, 95% CI 0.60–0.89). [23]

Originally Neo-Kiss was established on a voluntary participation basis, but since 2005 it became mandatory for all German neonatal units. This experience in using Neo-Kiss surveillance system indicates that it should focus on the most vulnerable infants, those of VLGA/VLBW and shows that only its implementation is able to significantly reduce HAI rates, possibly conditioned by standardizing definitions and by the feedback process established within the system. [24]For all above mentioned reasons, for its simplicity and sustainability, Neo-Kiss [23,24] has been proposed as a monitoring system at European level, and EuroNeoNet has decided to implement it in NICUs affiliated to the network. [15]

However, it is well recognized that information, by itself, is not sufficient to produce improvements in care, if it is not translated into changes in clinical practice in order to improve outcomes. Models currently used for prevention of infection are evidence-based and combine interventions with built-in continuous quality improvement initiatives. These models exemplify the integration of results of clinical research into daily clinical practice, aiming to provide high quality care, focused on systems that tend to be error-free in the implementation of effective change and to assessing its impact. [32]

Strategies to Prevent HAI in Neonatal Intensive Care

The scientific evidence confirms HAI is potentially preventable, the estimated avoidable proportion being between 10 and 70%, depending on the setting, baseline infection rate and type of infections [23,24]. However, achieving a zero sepsis rate in neonates seems to be an almost impossible goal. [33] In adults, Haley et al [25] showed that with a minimal effort, infection rate could be reduced by 6% and the implementation of a specific control program could achieve a 32% reduction.

> It is evident from previous experiences that prevention of HAI in newborn infants is possible but not an easy task. It is necessary to implement a standardised easy-to-use surveillance system, as well as long-term well constructed intervention strategies, based on reliable scientific evidence that considers the multiple factors involved in HAI pathogenesis (hands of health workers, presence of vascular catheters and endotracheal intubation).
>
> The Institute of Medicine 2001 report “Crossing the Quality Chasm” outlined the six characteristics to be offered by health systems: safe, effective, efficient, patient centered timely and equitable care. So, the concept of Patient Safety is now embedded in health care, and is generally approached by voluntary reporting systems of adverse events. However, HAI being a clear case of break in safety is not usually approached this way but rather by implementing evidence-based good and safe clinical practices.

Several groups developed neonatal experimental studies and randomized clinical trials to evaluate several strategies aimed to prevent HAI. These combined interventions basically consisted of recollection and diffusion of scientific evidence and the simultaneous application of a set of preventive measures along with the establishment of an environment of intense multidisciplinary collaboration, to design and develop plans to improve the quality of care for patients. [15,17,24,34,35]

Based on this philosophy, the Canadian Neonatal Network (CNN), demonstrated a reduction of both, HAI and Chronic Lung Disease. This study also found that intervention directed towards a specific outcome may affect others so they propose to apply interventions aiming at multiple outcomes. [35] Likewise, by exploring the opinion of health care professionals, CNN has identified individual and institutional factors to facilitate or not allow changes in medical practice. So these institutional elements must be considered to design strategies for health care improvement.

All these experiences indicate that HAI prevention in neonates continues to present an elusive target that requires a big and multi-disciplinary approach. It is necessary to develop a well-constructed and continuous effort, based on reliable scientific evidence that considers the multiple factors involved in the transmission of HAI. However it is essential to establish surveillance systems and intervention strategies of proven clinical efficacy that have been appropriately evaluated by well designed large randomised clinical trials.

Specific Preventive Measures to Be Implemented

In newborn infants, much like in older children and adults, HAI is associated with three main risk factors, improper hand-washing, use of intravascular catheters and intubation and mechanical ventilation. Lists of potentially better practices for prevention of HAI in neonates are available. [17, 36]

Hand washing. Frequent hand-washing with an appropriate technique is the easiest, less expensive and most effective strategy. However, hand-washing has effectively been replaced by hand rubbing with alcohol-based waterless gels, because of their rapid bactericidal action, broad antimicrobial effect, readiness of use and rapid evaporation, as long as hands are not soiled with organic matter. [37] It is estimated that at least one third of all HAI could be avoided with good hand hygiene. But promotion of hand hygiene is one of the major challenges for all health systems, because many individual and institutional factors have been linked to the difficulties in its implementation. [25]

Catheter-related infections. Probably, the most important measure is the daily evaluation of the risks and benefits of maintaining catheters in place [38]. The application of strict measures for catheter insertion and maintenance, ideally performed by a dedicated team, reduces by a third the risk of blood stream infection in VLBW infants.[39] Also, several manoeuvres to decrease catheter-related infections have been proposed, like subcutaneous tunnelled catheters, use of sponges impregnated with chlorhexidine or antibiotics [40,41] or vancomycin flushes. [42]

Endotracheal intubation and mechanical ventilation. Its use is associated with a reduction in neonatal mortality but an increase in infections. [43,44] Recommended measures to prevent infections range from hand-washing, use of disposable gloves and close-tracheal aspiration systems. [42] Nasal continuous positive pressure support is widely used to avoid the need for intubation, [45] to facilitate early extubation and to prevent the need for reintubation. [46] Recently, noninvasive nasal ventilation has been introduced in VLBW infants to further prevent need for tracheal intubation. [47]

It is important to highlight that many of other measures proposed for HAI prevention have not been evaluated in neonates, and thus might not be effective. An example of this is the use of chlorhexidine for vaginal disinfection and newborn's skin care [48,49] or that of catheter impregnation with antiseptics or antibiotics [41,50,51], that seem promising but need more research to establish their safety. [40,41]

We must not forget the terrible consequences of the generalized use in the sixties of hexachlorophene bathing to prevent *Staphylococcus aureus* skin colonization, It was eventually proven not only ineffective but promoted gram negative colonization. [52] More importantly, it caused neurotoxicity producing in premature infants a vacuolar spongiphorme encephalopathy from the brainstem reticular formation [53] since it was absorbed through the skin. [54] This type of experience must never happen again.

How to Best Implement These Preventive Measures?

It is well recognized that just knowing what to do to prevent HAI and taking the decision to implement that knowledge, is not enough to decrease the rates of HAI. The key issue is not *WHAT TO DO,* but rather *HOW TO DO IT.* Clinicians should not rely only on knowledge of the evidence-based preventive measures required to decrease HAI and on the willingness of health professionals to implement them, but should use quality improvement methodologies developed by implementation sciences. Although it is not within the scope of this article to review in detail these methodologies, a few paragraphs are included with the key facts about them. For readers interested in learning more about them, relevant references are provided.

Making improvements in health services requires changes and changes can be threatening or overwhelming for busy NICU personnel. It is obvious that while every improvement involves changes, not every change is an improvement. Making changes to the way that we do things can be time-consuming and can sometimes feel risky. To overcome these difficulties, health services implementation researchers have developed theoretical models for changes applying different methods [55], considering existing barriers and using trained facilitators to make the chances happen to improve the quality of care provided. Quality improvement involves prospective and retrospective reviews to improve and measure where we are, and finding ways to make it better. It avoids attributing blame and creates systems to prevent errors, trying to find where the system "defect" is. There is plenty of evidence that it is highly effective. The model provides a framework for developing, testing and implementing changes to the way that things are done that will lead to improvement.

When applied to health care, quality improvements means "the combined and increasing efforts of healthcare professionals, researchers, patients and their families, payers, planners and educators to make changes leading to better patient outcomes, system performance (care) and professional development." [56]

The basic quality improvement model is the so-call *PDSA-cycle bundle* method (see: www.ihi.org/ihi/topics/improvement/improvementmethods/) It consists of setting up a project team to define the goals (reduction of HAI), design evidence-based projects (*Plan*), implement them (*Do*), and finally measure the effects of their actions (*Study*). If needed, other quality improvement actions (*Act*) are started in new quality improvement bundles. The key to PDSA cycles is to try out changes on a small scale to begin with and to rely on using many consecutive cycles to build up information about how effective your change is.

To establish a successful program to prevent HAI, the use of the Plan-Do-Study-Act-cycle multiple bundle methodology is strongly recommended, as it has been shown to be effective. [57] It must also be based on evidence, team learning and acting, and above all on a culture for patient safety. To implement such a preventive strategy, the following key action steps are suggested:

Plan

1. Set up a small multidisciplinary working team for improvement with a strong leadership, including at least a neonatologist, a neonatal nurse, a microbiologist and a hospital administrator. The addition of an expert in quality improvement as a facilitator is strongly recommended to enhance the chances of success of the preventive plan.
2. Select and implement a neonatal surveillance system to measure and compare the incidence of HAI, like the NEO-KISS.
3. Identify the evidence-based preventive measures shown effective in neonates.
4. Select those recommendations not already fully implemented in the NICU.
5. Quantify and prioritize them according to their expected impact and difficulty to be implemented, and select those to be used.

Do

1. After identifying the evidence-based recommendations to be implemented, select a few quality improvement projects, perhaps in key areas such as hand-hygiene and catheter management and develop few indicators easy to collect.
2. Disseminate the preventive plans among all health professionals of the NICU to assure their full knowledge and understanding, and stimulate their proactive participation for their full implementation.
3. Periodically measure the rate of implementation of the recommendations selected (process indicators), as well as their effect on the rate of HAI episodes (outcome indicators).

Study

1. Periodically analyse and provide feedback of the project´s results and achievements, stressing the positive results and correcting the negative ones.
2. Assure the sustainability of the program by making all interested parties, health professionals, hospital administrators and parents, aware of the impact of the preventive measures on their main area of interest, improvement in the quality of care provided, economic savings, and long term benefits for infants, families, and the society as a whole.

Act

1. Redefine procedures to solve any deviations from the original plan or not fully accomplished.
2. Initiate new quality improvement projects to further decrease the incidence of HAI, with the ideal final target a "*sepsis cero rate*", however unachievable.

Summary and Recommendations

In summary, neonatal sepsis is a frequent and severe condition that increases mortality as well as short and long term morbidities, especially affecting growth and neurodevelopment. The difficulties of establishing an early diagnosis impede prescribing appropriate treatment. Thus, a high index of suspicion must be present at all times, and efforts must be concentrated on its prevention. Neonatal HAI is potentially preventable by using a few proven not expensive interventions, like a good hand hygiene technique and rational use and adherence to protocols for catheter placement and maintenance. However, the full implementation of these recommendations is not an easy task.

Participation in a neonatal network for benchmarking although useful, is not enough to assure a sustained decrease in the HAI incidence, to the lowest levels achieved by some NICUs. The implementation of a specific neonatal HAI surveillance system, to be implemented for at least all VLGA infants at highest risk for severe HAI, is strongly recommended. The use of the PDSA-cycle bundled multiple intervention method and establishment of a quality improvement team for change, to lead, design, supervise and implement the evidence-based and safe selected preventive practices in the NICU is the key to success.

Acknowledgment

We like to thank Jose I. Pijoan, Jose I. Villate, and Mikel Latorre for their expert advice and to Elizabeth Valls for her technical assistance in preparing the manuscript.

Authors have no conflict of interest to disclose.

References

[1] Vergnano S, Sharland M, Kazembe P, Mwansambo C, Heath PT. Neonatal Sepsis: an international perspective. *Arch. Dis. Child Fetal Neonatal.* Ed. 2005;90:F220-F224.

[2] Zaidi AK, Huskins WC, Thaver D, et al. Hospital-acquired neonatal infections in developing countries. *Lancet.* 2005;365:1175–88.

[3] Stoll BJ. Neonatal infections: a global perspective. In: Remington JS, Klein JO, eds. *Infectious Diseases of the Fetus and Newborn Infant.* 6th ed. Philadelphia, PA: WB Saunders; 2005;27–57.

[4] Baker CJ. Nosocomial septicemia and meningitis in neonates. *Am. J. Med.* 1981;70:698-701.

[5] Phillips P, Cortina-Borja M, Millar M, Gilbert R. Risk-adjusted surveillance of hospital-acquired infections in neonatal intensive care units: a systematic review. *J. Hosp. Infect.* 2008;Nov;70(3):203-11.

[6] Lopez Sastre JB, Coto CD, Fernandez CB. Neonatal sepsis of nosocomial origin: an epidemiological study from the "Grupo de Hospitales Castrillo". *J. Perinat. Med.* 2002;30(2):149-57.

[7] Stoll BJ, Hansen N. Infections in VLBW infants: studies from the NICHD Neonatal Research Network. *Semin. Perinatol.* 2003;Aug;27(4):293-301.

[8] March of Dimes, PMNCH, Save the Children, WHO. In: Howson CP, Kinney MV,Lawn JE, eds. Born too soon: the global action report on preterm birth. Geneva: World Health Organization, 2012.

[9] Harvey, David (David Robert) and De Louvois, John Infection in the newborn. Wiley, Chichester, West Sussex, England ; New York, 1990.

[10] Stoll BJ, Hansen NI, Adams-Chapman I, Fanaroff AA, Hintz SR, Vohr B, et al., Neurodevelopmental and growth impairment among extremely low-birth-weight infants with neonatal infection. *JAMA.* 2004;292:2357-65.

[11] Schlapbach LJ, Aebischer M, Adams M, Natalucci G, Bonhoeffer J, Latzin P, et al. Impact of sepsis on neurodevelopmental outcome in a Swiss National Cohort of extremely premature infants. *Pediatrics.*2011; Aug;128(2):e348-e357.

[12] Johnson TJ, Patel AL, Jegier BJ, Engstrom JL, Meier PP. Cost of Morbidities in Very Low Birth Weight Infants. *J. Pediatr.* 2012; Aug 18.

[13] Kaplan HC, Lannon C, Walsh MC, Donovan EF. Ohio Statewide Quality-Improvement Collaborative to Reduce Late-Onset Sepsis in Preterm Infants. *Pediatrics.* 2011; Feb 21.

[14] Kruse M, Michelsen SI, Flachs EM, Bronnum-Hansen H, Madsen M, Uldall P. Lifetime costs of cerebral palsy. *Dev. Med. Child Neurol.* 2009; Aug;51(8):622-8.

[15] Soler A, Madrid M, Geffers C, Hummler HD. International Perspectives: Preventing Sepsis in VLBW Infants: Experience from Neonatal Networks and Voluntary Surveillance Systems. *NeoReviews.* 2010; Aug 1;11(8):e403-e408.

[16] Haque KN. Definitions of bloodstream infection in the newborn. *Pediatr. Crit. Care Med.* 2005;6:S45-S49.

[17] Horbar JD, Rogowski J, Plsek PE, Delmore P, Edwards WH, Hocker J, et al. Collaborative quality improvement for neonatal intensive care. NIC/Q Project Investigators of the Vermont Oxford Network. *Pediatrics.* 2001;Jan;107(1):14-22.

[18] Neal PR, Kleiman MB, Reynolds JK, Allen SD, Lemons JA, Yu PL. Volume of blood submitted for culture from neonates. *J. Clin. Microbiol.* 1986;24:353-6.

[19] Schelonka RL, Chai MK, Yoder BA, Hensley D, Brockett RM, Ascher DP. Volume of blood required to detect common neonatal pathogens. *J. Pediatr.* 1996;129:275-8.

[20] European Medicine Agency[http://www.ema.europa.eu/docs/en_ GB/document_ library/Report/2010/12/WC500100199.pdf]. London: Report on the Expert meeting on Neonatal and Paediatric Sepsis EMA/477725/2010. 2010. [accessed August 2013].

[21] Horan TC, Andrus M, Dudeck MA. CDC/NHSN surveillance definition of health care-associated infection and criteria for specific types of infections in the acute care setting. *Am. J. Infect. Control.* 2008;36:309-32.

[22] Vincent JL, Opal SM, Marshall JC, Tracey KJ. Sepsis definitions: time for change. *Lancet.* 2013;381:774-5.

[23] Geffers C, Baerwolff S, Schwab F, Gastmeier P. Incidence of healthcare-associated infections in high-risk neonates: results from the German surveillance system for very-low-birthweight infants. *J. Hosp. Infect.* 2008;Mar;68(3):214-21.

[24] Schwab F, Geffers C, Barwolff S, Ruden H, Gastmeier P. Reducing neonatal nosocomial bloodstream infections through participation in a national surveillance system. *J. Hosp. Infect.* 2007; Apr;65(4):319-25.

[25] Haley RW, Culver DH, White JW, Morgan WM, Emori TG, Munn VP, et al. The efficacy of infection surveillance and control programs in preventing nosocomial infections in US hospitals. *Am. J. Epidemiol.*1985;Feb;121(2):182-205.

[26] Valls A, Halliday HL, Hummler H. International Perspectives: Neonatal Networking: A European Perspective. *NeoReviews.*2007;Jul 1;8(7):e275-e281.

[27] Vergnano S, Menson E, Kennea N, Embleton N, Russell AB, Watts T, et al. Neonatal infections in England: the NeonIN surveillance network. *Archives of Disease in Childhood* - Fetal and Neonatal Edition. 2011;Jan 1;96(1):F9-F14.

[28] Couto RC, Pedrosa TM, Tofani CP, Pedroso ER. Risk factors for nosocomial infection in a neonatal intensive care unit. *Infect. Control. Hosp. Epidemiol.* 2006;27:571-5.

[29] Coello R, Gastmeier P, de Boer AS. Surveillance of hospital-acquired infection in England, Germany, and The Netherlands: will international comparison of rates be possible? *Infect. Control. Hosp. Epidemiol.* 2001; Jun;22(6):393-7.

[30] Schwab F, Gastmeier P, Piening B, Geffers C. The step from a voluntary to a mandatory national nosocomial infection surveillance system: the influence on infection rates and surveillance effect. *Antimicrob. Resist. Infect. Control.* 2012;1(1):24.

[31] Gastmeier P, Hentschel J, de Veer I,Obladen M, Ruden H. Device-associated nosocomial infection surveillance in neonatal intensive care using specified criteria for neonates. *J. Hosp. Infect.*1998;38:51–60.

[32] Bishop-Kurylo D. The clinical experience of continuous quality improvement in the neonatal intensive care unit. *J. Perinat. Neonatal Nurs.*1998;12:51-7.

[33] McKee C, Berkowitz I, Cosgrove SE, Bradley K, Beers C, Perl TM, et al. Reduction of catheter-associated bloodstream infections in pediatric patients: experimentation and reality. *Pediatr. Crit. Care Med.* 2008;Jan;9(1):40-6.

[34] Lee SK, Aziz K, Singhal N, Cronin CM, James A, Lee DS, et al. Improving the quality of care for infants: a cluster randomized controlled trial. *CMAJ.*2009;Oct 13;181(8):469-76.

[35] Stevens B, Lee SK, Law MP, Yamada J. A qualitative examination of changing practice in Canadian neonatal intensive care units. *J. Eval. Clin. Pract.* 2007; Apr;13(2):287-94.

[36] Powers RJ, Wirtschafter DW. Decreasing central line associated bloodstream infection in neonatal intensive care. *Clin. Perinatol.*2010;37:247-72.

[37] Pittet D. Improving adherence to hand hygiene practice: a multidisciplinary approach. *Emerg. Infect. Dis.*2001; 7:234-40.

[38] American Academy of Pediatrics, The American College of Obstetricians and Gynecologist. Infection Control. In: American Academy of Pediatrics, The American

College of Obstetricians and Gynecologist, editors. *Guidelines for Perinatal Care.* Sixth ed. 2007.p.349-70.

[39] Maas A, Flament P, Pardou A, Deplano A, Dramaix M, Struelens MJ. Central venous catheter-related bacteraemia in critically ill neonates: risk factors and impact of a prevention programme. *J. Hosp. Infect.*1998;40:211-24.

[40] Veenstra DL, Saint S, Sullivan SD. Cost-effectiveness of antiseptic-impregnated central venous catheters for the prevention of catheter-related bloodstream infection. *JAMA*.1999;282:554-60.

[41] Lee OK, Johnston L. A systematic review for effective management of central venous catheters and catheter sites in acute care paediatric patients. *Worldviews Evid Based Nurs.*2005;2:4-13.

[42] Jarvis WR. The United States approach to strategies in the battle against healthcare-associated infections, 2006: transitioning from benchmarking to zero tolerance and clinician accountability. *Journal of Hospital Infection*. 2007;65:3-9.

[43] Henderson Smart David J , Wilkinson Andrew R , Raynes Greenow Camille H Mechanical ventilation for newborn infants with respiratory failure due to pulmonary disease Cochrane Database of Systematic Reviews : Reviews 2002 Issue 4 John Wiley & Sons , Ltd C. 2002.

[44] Spence Kaye , Barr Peter Nasal versus oral intubation for mechanical ventilation of newborn infants Cochrane Database of Systematic Reviews : Reviews 1999 Issue 2 John Wiley & Sons , Ltd Chichester, UK DOI : 10 1002 /14651858 CD000948. 1999.

[45] Subramaniam P, Henderson-Smart DJ, Davis PG. Prophylactic nasal continuous positive airways pressure for preventing morbidity and mortality in very preterm infants. *Cochrane Database Syst. Rev.* 2005;CD001243.

[46] Davis PG, Henderson-Smart DJ. Nasal continuous positive airways pressure immediately after extubation for preventing morbidity in preterm infants. *Cochrane Database Syst. Rev.* 2003;CD000143.

[47] Sai Sunil KM, Dutta S, Kumar P. Early nasal intermittent positive pressure ventilation versus continuous positive airway pressure for respiratory distress syndrome. *Acta Paediatr.* 2009;98:1412-5.

[48] Upadhyayula S, Kambalapalli M, Harrison CJ. Safety of anti-infective agents for skin preparation in premature infants. *Arch. Dis. Child.* 2007;92:646-7.

[49] Stade B, Shah V, Ohlsson A. Vaginal chlorhexidine during labour to prevent early-onset neonatal group B streptococcal infection. *Cochrane Database Syst. Rev.* 2004;CD003520.

[50] Chien LY, Macnab Y, Aziz K, Andrews W, McMillan DD, Lee SK. Variations in central venous catheter-related infection risks among Canadian neonatal intensive care units. *Pediatr. Infect. Dis. J.* 2002;21:505-511.

[51] Shah PS, Shah N. Heparin-bonded catheters for prolonging the patency of central venous catheters in children. *Cochrane Database Syst Rev.* 2007;CD005983.

[52] Light IJ, Sutherland JM. What is the evidence that hexachlorophene is not effective? *Pediatrics.*1973;51:345-349.

[53] Shuman RM, Leech RW, Alvord EC, Jr. Neurotoxicity of hexachlorophene in the human: I. A clinicopathologic study of 248 children. *Pediatrics.*1974;54:689-95.

[54] Kopelman AE. Cutaneous absorption of hexachlorophene in low-birth-weight infants. *J. Pediatr.*1973;82:972-975.

[55] Payne NR, Carpenter JH, Badger GJ, Horbar JD, Rogowski J. Marginal increase in cost and excess length of stay associated with nosocomial bloodstream infections in surviving very low birth weight infants.*Pediatrics*.2004; Aug;114(2):348-55.

[56] Batalden PB, Davidoff F. What is "quality improvement" and how can it transform healthcare? *Qual. Saf. Health Care*.2007;Feb;16(1):2-3.

[57] Sawyer M, Weeks K, Goeschel CA, Thompson DA, Berenholtz SM, Marsteller JA, et al. Using evidence, rigorous measurement, and collaboration to eliminate central catheter-associated bloodstream infections. *Crit. Care Med.*2010;38:S292-S298.

In: Sepsis
Editor: Nancy Khardori

ISBN: 978-1-63117-244-1

Chapter 5

Sepsis in Adults: Risk Factors, Diagnosis, Management and Health Outcomes

Suma S. Rao[1,2], M.D., A. S. M. M. Akther[3], MRCP., and Nancy Khardori[4,5], M.D., Ph.D.

[1]Infectious Diseases, Changi General Hospital, Singapore
[2]Internal Medicine, Changi General Hospital, Singapore
[3]Division of Infectious Diseases, Department of Internal Medicine, and , Department of Microbiology and Molecular cell Biology, Eastern Virginia medical School, Norfolk, Virginia, US
[4]Division of Infectious Diseases, Department of Internal Medicine, Eastern Virginia Medical School, Norfolk, Virginia, US
[5]Professor, Department of Microbiology and Molecular cell Biology, Eastern Virginia medical School, Norfolk, Virginia, US

Abstract

Sepsis, the syndrome caused by systemic inflammatory response to infection remains a major cause of morbidity and mortality in adults. Patients become septic following a major break in host defenses that increases the likelihood of infection. The incidence of sepsis increases with age, is higher in men, African Americans and other nonwhites and in patients with comorbidities. Elderly patients with sepsis comprise an increasing proportion of intensive care unit admissions with a considerably higher risk of dying. A number of disorders including acute myocardial infarction, acute pancreatitis, and diabetic ketoacidosis mimic the clinical presentation of sepsis. Therefore, for early diagnosis, it is necessary to recognize historical, clinical and laboratory findings that indicate infection, organ dysfunction and global tissue hypoxia. Blood culture positivity increases with greater volume of blood used rather timing or use of multiple sites. However, negative blood cultures do not rule out the presence of septicemia and sepsis. Urine cultures and other site specific cultures may help in the microbiological diagnosis of sepsis infection. The biomarkers currently available are not reliable for diagnosis. Procalcitonin may be better employed to rule out rather than make a diagnosis of sepsis especially if multiple measurements over time are used. Management of sepsis includes hemodynamic resuscitation, ventilatory support and early and aggressive antimicrobial therapy. Surviving sepsis campaign recommends initiating antibiotic therapy within the first hour of recognition of the potential diagnosis after appropriate cultures have been obtained. Control of the infection process at the source is critical to the outcome as is organ system focused antimicrobial therapy especially in patients with negative blood cultures. The usefulness of antagonists of cytokine cascade has been under intense investigation, but none has proven to be effective and safe at the time of this writing.

Sepsis and septic shock persist as major healthcare problems despite on-going research to improve outcomes. Overall mortality from severe sepsis or septic shock still is30-60% despite aggressive medical care. Sepsis is the 10th leading cause of death in the United States and cost 14.6 billion dollars in expenditure in 2008. Sepsis syndrome results from a host reaction to infection, including a robust systemic inflammatory response, enhanced coagulation and impaired fibrinolysis. The cause of death in sepsis usually is multi-organ failure.

The systemic inflammatory response syndrome (SIRS) is defined by the constellation of fever or hypothermia, tachycardia, tachypnea and leucocytosis or leucopenia, or the presence of immature neutrophils. SIRS can result from numerous conditions but only becomes “sepsis” when infection is the inciting cause. The terms severe sepsis and sepsis are used interchangeably.

Term	Definition and Criteria
Infection	Microorganism invasion of a normally sterile site
Bacteremia	Presence of viable microorganisms in the blood
Systemic Inflammatory Response Syndrome (SIRS)	A systemic inflammatory response to a pathologic insult, such as a burn, trauma, pancreatitis, or infection. SIRS requires two or more of the following conditions: • Temperature >38 degree C or <36 degree C • Heart rate >90 beats/min • Respiratory rate >20 breaths/min or PaCO2 <32 mm Hg • WBC >12,000/mm3, <4000 cells/mm3, or >10% immature (band) forms
Sepsis	The syndrome caused by a systemic inflammatory response secondary to infection
Severe sepsis	Sepsis associated with organ dysfunction. Specific organ dysfunctions include, but are not limited to, hypotension, renal dysfunction, respiratory failure, and altered mental status.
Septic shock	Sepsis with hypotension or hypoperfusion despite adequate fluid resuscitation.
Hypotension, sepsis-induced	A decrease in systolic blood pressure <90 mm Hg, a mean arterial pressure <60 mm Hg, or a reduction of >40 mm Hg from baseline

Adapted from Bone RC, Balk RA, Cerra FB, et al. American-College of Chest Physicians Society of Critical Care Medicine Consensus Conference—definitions for sepsis and organ failure and guidelines for the use of innovative therapies in sepsis. Crit. Care Med. 1992;20(6):864–74.

Figure 1. Definitions related to Sepsis.

Epidemiology

The annual incidence of severe sepsis in several industrialized nations has been reported to be 50–100 cases per 100,000 persons [1]. The rate of hospitalisation secondary to severe sepsis is increasing even faster than predicted [2]. In the United States, the number of hospitalizations for severe sepsis per 100,000 persons increased from 143 in 2000 to 343 in 2007. The mean length of hospital stay decreased from 17.3 to 14.9 days. The mortality rate decreased from 39% to 27% [3].

There are also age, sex and racial differences in the incidence of sepsis. The incidence of sepsis disproportionately increases with advancing age (age >65 years), which is also an independent predictor of mortality [4]. Respiratory infections are the most common cause of sepsis in elderly. [4].Men have higher incidence than women for all sources of sepsis except genitourinary tract [5, 6]. African Americans and other non-whites have higher incidences of sepsis for all sources of sepsis. Racial differences in severe sepsis can be explained by both a higher infection rate and a higher risk of acute organ dysfunction in black compared to white individuals [7].Sepsis incidence, race and sex differences are present in the distribution of several common co-morbid conditions, including alcohol abuse, diabetes, HIV, end-stage renal failure, and cancer. For example, African Americans and non-white patients with sepsis are more likely to have several concurrent diagnoses that are associated with an increased risk of infection, including diabetes, end-stage renal disease, HIV, and alcohol abuse. Similarly, male patients with sepsis are more likely to have obstructive pulmonary disease, cancer, alcohol abuse, or HIV than female patients with sepsis [8].

Risk Factors for Sepsis in Adults

Patients do not become septic without a major breach in host defences that increases the likelihood of infection. Important host factors include access to appropriate healthcare, age, nutrition and the presence of comorbid illnesses that can modify the response of the immune system to infection or increase the risk of acute organ failure. Patients with diabetes mellitus have an increased risk of developing infections and sepsis and are more likely to develop renal failure during the course of sepsis [9, 10].

Elderly patients comprise an increasing proportion of intensive care unit (ICU) admissions. The risk of dying from severe sepsis is considerably higher in the elderly and very elderly subgroup of patients, with age as an independent risk factor for mortality [11]. Age, cancer chemotherapy, immunosuppressive medications, chronic illness, alcoholism and major organ surgery are known to suppress the immune system predisposing to sepsis. Sepsis itself can cause immunosuppression. Patients who die in the ICU following sepsis compared with patients who die of non-sepsis etiologies were found to have biochemical, flow cytometric, and immunohistochemical findings consistent with immunosuppression [12]. Chronic alcohol abuse is associated with a persistent fever, delayed resolution of symptoms, increased rates of bacteremia, increased use of intensive care, prolonged duration of hospital stay, and increased cost of hospitalization for infected patients. Sepsis is associated with a reduced quality of life in those who survive their acute illness [8].Genetic variability also plays a role in determining susceptibility and outcome of infection [13].

Surgical patients are vulnerable to infectious complications during hospitalization. Incidence of infectious complications mostly depends on type of wound, urgent or elective surgery, site of surgery and use of prosthetic material. Severe sepsis and organ failure are major causes of postoperative morbidity and mortality after large visceral surgery [14].

In hospitalized patients, presence of Intravenous cannulas/central lines , urinary catheters, long duration of hospitalization, intensive care unit admission, presence of innate virulent and resistant pathogens are independent risk factors for development of sepsis.

Disorders That Mimic Sepsis

A significant number of patients identified with a sepsis syndrome at presentation are eventually diagnosed as having non-infectious diseases although clinical characteristics of these patients are similar to those of patients with culture-positive sepsis [15].

Mimics of sepsis should be recognized to treat the condition and to avoid inappropriate treatment with antibiotics. Disorders that mimic sepsis include acute myocardial infarction, inflammatory colitis, medication effects i.e., diuretic-induced hypovolemia, relative adrenal insufficiency, inadequate steroid therapy, acute pulmonary embolus, gastrointestinal haemorrhage, acute pancreatitis, diabetic ketoacidosis, systemic lupus erythematosus flare and rectus sheath hematoma.

Diagnosis of Sepsis Syndrome

To diagnose severe sepsis/septic shock as early as possible, it is necessary to recognize historical, clinical and laboratory findings that are indicative of infection, organ dysfunction and global tissue hypoxia. General clinical signs like fever, chills, and hypotension are nonspecific. However, a complete physical exam often reveals an obvious or occult local source of infection. Presence of a urinary catheter or vascular catheter implicate them as the sources of sepsis.

The laboratory tests used in the diagnosis of sepsis include a complete blood cell count with differential (CBC), standard chemistry panel, including bicarbonate and creatinine; liver enzymes; lactate level and coagulation studies. Clinicians have traditionally relied on leukocytosis, neutrophilia and bandemia as indicators of bacterial etiology and as a measure of the severity of illness. However, these indicators have poor accuracy and thus cannot be used alone to either exclude or confirm the diagnosis of bacterial infection [16, 17, 18]. Overwhelming sepsis can also be associated with leucopenia and neutropenia. CBC may also reveal hemo-concentration with raised hemoglobin and hematocrit because of significant hypovolemia.

Thrombocytopenia is an independent predictor of multiple organ failure and poor outcome [19]. Lactic acid levels are increasingly being employed to screen for global tissue hypoxia [20]. Of note, hyperlactatemia is not always accompanied by a low bicarbonate level and/or elevated anion gap, and thus, a lactate level should be considered if severe sepsis is suspected. An arterial or central venous sample should be sent for assessing lactate levels, particularly if peripheral venous lactate is elevated as sometimes peripheral lactate may be falsely elevated [21]. In a study of 1690 patients with sepsis, 99.7% of patients had a baseline elevated D-Dimer and 93.4% of patients had prolonged pro-thrombin time [22, 23]. Hence a work-up for disseminated intravascular coagulation (DIC) is suggested if severe sepsis or septic shock is suspected.

Severe sepsis definition = sepsis-induced tissue hypoperfusion or organ dysfunction (any of the following thought to be due to the infection)
Sepsis-induced hypotension
Lactate above upper limits laboratory normal
Urine output < 0.5 mL/kg/hr for more than 2 hrs despite adequate fluid resuscitation
Acute lung injury with Pa_{O_2}/Fi_{O_2} < 250 in the absence of pneumonia as infection source
Acute lung injury with Pa_{O_2}/Fi_{O_2} < 200 in the presence of pneumonia as infection source
Creatinine > 2.0 mg/dL (176.8 μmol/L)
Bilirubin > 2 mg/dL (34.2 μmol/L)
Platelet count < 100,000 μL
Coagulopathy (international normalized ratio > 1.5)

Source: Levy MM, Fink MP, Marshall JC, et al: 2001 SCCM/ESICM/ACCP/ATS/SIS International Sepsis Definitions Conference. Crit Care Med 2003; 31: 1250–1256.

Figure 2.

Appropriate cultures should be obtained before antimicrobial treatment if such cultures do not cause significant delay (>45 minutes) in administration of antibiotics. The recommended practice is to culture at or above 20ml of blood divided evenly into aerobic and anaerobic bottles. Blood cultures should not be drawn through an intravenous catheter at the time of catheter insertion. Doing so increases the false positive rate of the blood culture [24]. In the presence of an indwelling catheter (for more than 48 hours), at least one set should be drawn through each lumen. Also, there is no difference in the yield whether blood samples for cultures are drawn simultaneously or at intervals within a 24 hour period [25]. Hence at least two pairs of blood cultures should be obtained in a patient being evaluated for severe sepsis/septic shock. For rapid identification of bacterial species from positive blood cultures DNA-based microarray platform was found to have high sensitivity, specificity, and was faster than the gold-standard culture-based method [26].

Blood culture yield increases with greater blood volume obtained and volume appears to be more important than timing or use of multiple sites. In two studies evaluating yield for four or more blood cultures (volume 20 mL), the cumulative yield for true pathogens increased with the first (73-80%), second (80-89%), third (95-98%) and fourth (99-100%) of cultures collected [27, 28]. However, in another study, the yield from two blood cultures (30 mL in each of two bottles) was the same as the yield from three blood cultures (20 mL in each of three bottles) [29]. One blood culture set is rarely advisable or sufficient. A single blood culture lacks sensitivity as well as precludes the ability to distinguish contaminants from true bacteremia with bacteria that are common contaminants like coagulase negative staphylococci and diphtheroids [30]. Fever at the time of blood culture collection is not specific or sensitive for the presence of bacteremia [25].

Contamination of blood culture can occur even when precise techniques for collection and processing are used. However, Staphylococcus aureus, Streptococcus pneumoniae, Group A Streptococci, Enterobacteriaceae, Hemophilus influenzae, Pseudomonas aeruginosa, Bacteroides and Candida species are always significant clinical pathogens and should not be regarded as contaminants, even in a single culture.

Urine cultures are appropriate in most patients unless there is an obvious alternate source and should always be coupled with urine analysis. Gram stain of urine sediment can give a clue as to the etiological agent in urinary infection. Gram stain and culture of sputum has low overall yield but is recommended for patients admitted to the ICU with pneumonia. Any purulent material from skin and soft-tissue infections and other normally sterile fluids should be obtained for gram stain and culture if there is evidence of localized infection. Testing pneumococcal and Legionella antigens in the urine is recommended for patients being admitted to the ICU and those with co-morbidities.

Rapid influenza antigen testing from nasopharyngeal swab is also recommended where deemed necessary. If invasive candidiasis is suspected, 1, 3 Beta-D- Glucan assay, mannan and anti-mannan antibody assays are suggested in addition to cultures.

Imaging studies such as chest x-ray, computed tomography (CT) scan of abdomen/pelvis etc., should be performed promptly in attempts to confirm a potential source of infection. However, patient risk from transportation and invasive procedures is an important consideration.

Use of Biomarkers in the Diagnosis of Sepsis

Multiple biological markers of sepsis including C-reactive protein(CRP), interleukin-6(IL-6), procalcitonin(PCT) and protein C have been investigated both for their diagnostic and prognostic capabilities. Bacteremic infections appear to cause the highest elevation in PCT with lower or negligible rises in localized bacterial, viral and intracellular bacterial infections [31, 32]. Gram-negative bacteremias seem to cause higher PCT rises than Gram-positive bacteremias [33]. Studies on procalcitonin are inconclusive about proving it as the single definitive test for the diagnosis of sepsis due to bacterial infections. A recent meta-analysis accounting for 3244 patients concluded that procalcitonin is a helpful marker for diagnosis of sepsis in critically ill patients, but that it must be interpreted in context with information from careful medical history, physical examination, and when feasible, microbiological assessment [34]. Procalcitonin may be better employed to rule out rather than rule in systemic sepsis particularly if repeated measures are used [34].

Management

Management of the septic patient starts as soon as the patient has a probable diagnosis of sepsis. Organising management into bundles of care has been shown to be associated with consistent and significant improvement in survival and antibiotic use [35, 36]. A ''bundle'' is a group of interventions related to a disease process that, when executed together, result in better outcomes than when implemented individually. The individual bundle elements are built upon evidence-based practices.

Initial Resuscitation: This comprises of a set of tasks to be completed for all patients within the first 6 h following the onset of severe sepsis. The Surviving Sepsis Campaign recommends intravenous fluids, along with antibiotics, vasopressors and inotropic agents and source control for the early management of septic shock [37]. Early goal-directed therapy provides significant benefits with respect to outcome in patients with severe sepsis and septic shock [38]. The Surviving Sepsis Campaign [37] targets central venous pressure (CVP), mean arterial pressure (MAP), serum lactate level and central venous oxygen saturation (ScvO2) as guides for resuscitation.

These measurements, achieved with fluid resuscitation and vasoactive medications, are guidelines for goals of resuscitation, and assist in decision-making. Goals during the first 6 hours of resuscitation suggested by Surviving sepsis campaign are to maintain Central venous pressure of 8–12 mm Hg, Mean arterial pressure of (MAP) ≥ 65 mm Hg, Urine output of ≥ 0.5 mL/kg/hour, Central venous (superior vena cava) or mixed venous oxygen saturation of 70% or 65% [37].

Mean Arterial Pressure (MAP) represents the proportion of time in systole and diastole. An approximation can be made for MAP from the systolic blood pressure (SBP) and diastolic blood pressure (DBP) i.e., MAP= [(2 DBP)+SBP]/3. MAP greater than or equal to 65 mm Hg is necessary to maintain perfusion pressure and adequate flow at the arteriolar level. At pressures below this, autoregulation can be dysfunctional in many tissue beds [39, 40].

Tissue hypoxia suggested by central venous oxygen saturation (ScVO2) or mixed venous oxygen saturation (SVO2) concentration is an early marker of sepsis or marginal circulation. Attainment of an ScvO2 of 70% has significant impact on survival. [41, 42]. Studies have shown a tendency for increased oxygen consumption with an increased tissue oxygen extraction during initial hypodynamic or normodynamic circulation in septic shock. Tissue oxygen saturation below 78% is associated with increased mortality [43].

Hyperlactatemia is associated with hypoperfusion. Baseline high serum lactate is associated with mortality independent of clinically apparent organ dysfunction and shock in patients admitted to the emergency department with severe sepsis [44]. Lactate clearance over the first 6 hours of sepsis presentation has been shown to have a significant association with pro-inflammation and anti-inflammation, coagulation, apoptosis, organ dysfunction, and mortality [45, 46]. In patients with hyperlactatemia, lactate-guided therapy significantly reduces hospital mortality [47].

In patients in the emergency department with a sepsis diagnosis, early lactate normalization during the first 6 h of resuscitation was the strongest independent predictor of survival [48]. Surviving sepsis campaign recommends targeting resuscitation to normalize lactate in patients with elevated levels.

Hemodynamic resuscitation with intravenous fluid forms the backbone of the care of the patient with septic shock. Patients with septic shock frequently present with depletion of intravascular volume. This occurs for a variety of reasons including decreased oral intake, vomiting, diarrhea, sweating, increased sensible and insensible losses. Further contributions to hypovolemia include a maldistributive defect with vasodilatation, peripheral blood pooling, extravasation of fluid into the interstitial space and increased capillary endothelial permeability [49, 50]. Circulatory signs of hypovolemia include tachycardia, capillary refill time >2 s, skin mottling, cool extremities, arterial hypotension , decreased renal perfusion manifested by concentrated urine.

SURVIVING SEPSIS CAMPAIGN BUNDLES

TO BE COMPLETED WITHIN 3 HOURS:
1) Measure lactate level
2) Obtain blood cultures prior to administration of antibiotics
3) Administer broad spectrum antibiotics
4) Administer 30 mL/kg crystalloid for hypotension or lactate ≥4mmol/L

TO BE COMPLETED WITHIN 6 HOURS:
5) Apply vasopressors (for hypotension that does not respond to initial fluid resuscitation) to maintain a mean arterial pressure (MAP) ≥ 65 mm Hg
6) In the event of persistent arterial hypotension despite volume resuscitation (septic shock) or initial lactate ≥4 mmol/L (36 mg/dL):
   - Measure central venous pressure (CVP)*
   - Measure central venous oxygen saturation ($Scvo_2$)*
7) Remeasure lactate if initial lactate was elevated*

*Targets for quantitative resuscitation included in the guidelines are CVP of ≥8 mm Hg, $Scvo_2$ of ≥70%, and normalization of lactate.

Source: Surviving Sepsis Campaign: International Guidelines for Management of Severe Sepsis and Septic Shock: 2012 Crit Care Med 2013; 41:580–637.

Figure 3.

During the initial evaluation of the hemodynamically unstable patient an initial fluid bolus is typically warranted to maintain organ perfusion and cardiac output. But it comes with the risk of fluid overload and potential adverse effects, especially on the lungs. There is increasing evidence that excessive volume administration can worsen outcome [51, 52, 53, 54]. So further attempts should be made at determining volume responsiveness [55]. The concept of volume responsiveness refers to the principle illustrated by the Frank-Starling curve, which demonstrates that increases in left ventricular end diastolic volume lead to increased stroke volume and to cardiac output, until a plateau. The goal for the clinician is to determine where on this curve the patient lies. If the patient lies on the 'steep' portion of the curve rather than the plateau, a fluid bolus may be beneficial. There are several tools for assessing volume status and volume responsiveness. Measures of fluid responsiveness commonly used are central venous pressure (CVP) or right atrial pressure, pulmonary artery wedge pressure (PAWP), ultrasound and echocardiographic assessment of intracardiac, vena caval diameters, left-ventricular end-diastolic area after a fluid challenge or passive leg raising [56].

Initial fluid challenge with a crystalloid should be given to patients with sepsis-induced tissue hypo-perfusion and suspicion of hypovolemia [37]. A fluid challenge should be distinguished from conventional fluid administration which offers quantitation of the cardiovascular response during volume infusion and prompt correction of fluid deficits. It is important to define the amount of fluid to be administered over a defined interval and to monitor the response of fluid challenge. More rapid administration and greater amounts of fluid may be needed in some patients. Fluid challenge technique should be applied wherein fluid administration is continued as long as there is hemodynamic improvement either based on dynamic (e.g., change in pulse pressure, stroke volume variation) or static (e.g., arterial pressure, heart rate) variables. The fluid management in early goal directed therapy is supported by studies showing that aggressively titrated early fluid administration is associated with modulation of inflammation, microcirculation function, and better outcomes [57].

The Saline versus Albumin Fluid Evaluation (SAFE) study indicated that albumin administration was safe and equally as effective as isotonic saline [58]. There is evidence suggesting that albumin reduces mortality when used as a resuscitation fluid for patients with sepsis [59]. Surviving sepsis guidelines suggest the use of albumin in the fluid resuscitation of severe sepsis and septic shock when patients require substantial amounts of crystalloids.

Despite the fact that colloids are able to reduce the amount of fluid required to reach haemodynamic stability, there are growing safety concerns regarding the effects of artificial colloids such as hydroxyethyl starch (HES) on renal function [60, 61]. Patients with severe sepsis who received fluid resuscitation with HES had an increased risk of death and were more likely to require renal-replacement therapy, as compared with those receiving isotonic saline [62, 63]. Surviving sepsis guidelines suggest against the use of hydroxyethyl starches as part of fluid resuscitation in severe sepsis and septic shock.

Acute circulatory failure during septic shock is characterized by decreased vascular tone and/or by low cardiac output. If a patient remains persistently hypotensive after optimization of preload, the subsequent goal of resuscitation protocols is the maintenance of perfusion pressure through the use of vasopressors and inotropic agents. Vasopressor therapy is initiated to target a mean arterial pressure (MAP) of 65 mm Hg. Norepinephrine is the first-line vasopressor used in septic shock. It acts by stimulating the α1-adrenergic receptors of peripheral arteries causing arterial vasoconstriction. This allows a rapid restoration of arterial pressure. Norepinephrine might also exert an inotropic effect through β1 receptors. Norepinephrine increases cardiac preload and cardiac index [64]. Meta-analysis has demonstrated the superiority of norepinephrine over dopamine in a critically ill population of patients with septic shock [65]. Additionally, dopamine was associated with an increased risk of arrhythmias [66, 67]. Dopamine is associated with a significant increase in the rate of death in patients with cardiogenic shock [68]. Surviving sepsis guidelines recommend norepinephrine as the first choice vasopressor [37]. Dopamine can be used as an alternative to norepinephrine only in patients who are at a low risk of tachyarrhythmias and absolute or relative bradycardia [37]. Epinephrine can be added to norepinephrine as an additional agent when needed to maintain adequate blood pressure [37].

Vasopressin is both a vasopressor and an antidiuretic hormone. Vasopressin mediates vasoconstriction via V1-receptor activation on vascular smooth muscle. Relative vasopressin deficiency is seen in approximately one-third of late septic shock patients [69]. Vasopressin enhances the sensitivity of the vasculature to other pressor agents [70]. Combined infusion of Vasopressin and norepinephrine can be used for treatment of catecholamine-resistant vasodilator shock. Patients receiving vasopressin with norepinephrine show significantly higher blood pressure, increased MAP, improved cardiac performance, and less norepinephrine requirement [71, 72]. Vasopressin can be added to norepinephrine to raise MAP or to reduce norepinephrine requirement [37].

Dobutamine is a synthetic catecholamine acting predominantly via Beta 1 and Beta 2 adrenoceptors and having few effects on alpha 1 receptors. Because of its positive chronotropic and inotropic effects, dobutamine increases heart rate and cardiac index. It was also shown to increase oxygen delivery index (DO2I) [73]. In patients with low cardiac output with adequate left ventricular filling pressure or elevated cardiac filling pressures and adequate mean arterial pressure, dobutamine infusion can be added to vasopressors [37]. All patients requiring vasopressors should have an arterial catheter placed as soon as practical if resources are available.

Antibiotics: Prompt institution of antimicrobial therapy that is active against the potential causative pathogen(s) after obtaining appropriate cultures is crucial in the treatment of patients with severe infections and sepsis. Initial presumptive anti-infective therapy consists of one or more drugs that have activity against all likely pathogens and that penetrate in adequate concentrations into tissues/fluids presumed to be the source of sepsis. Effective antimicrobial administration within the first hour of documented hypotension was shown to be associated with increased survival to hospital discharge in adult patients with septic shock [74]. Inadequate antimicrobial therapy at admission with sepsis is associated with excess mortality and increased length of stay [75]. Elapsed times from triage and qualification for early goal-directed therapy to administration of appropriate antimicrobials have been shown to be primary determinants of mortality in patients with severe sepsis and septic shock [76]. Surviving Sepsis Campaign recommends initiating antibiotic therapy within the first hour of recognition of severe sepsis, after suitable cultures have been obtained [37].

Corticosteroids: Despite more than five decades of study and debate, the role of corticosteroid treatment in patients with severe sepsis and septic shock remains controversial. It is established that severe sepsis results in a sustained pro-inflammatory state. Experimental and human studies have shown hydrocortisone can reverse the systemic inflammatory response, endothelial activation, and coagulation disorders secondary to an infection [77]. Moreover, at low doses, corticosteroids have been shown to improve rather than to suppress innate immunity in patients with septic shock [78]. Treatment with low-dose hydrocortisone accelerates shock reversal in early hyperdynamic septic shock. This was accompanied by reduced production of proinflammatory cytokines, suggesting both hemodynamic and immunomodulatory effects of steroid treatment [79]. But the Corticosteroid Therapy of Septic Shock (CORTICUS) study, showed no improvement in sepsis outcome in terms of mortality in a general population of patients with septic shock, although the median time to shock reversal was 2 to 3 days shorter in the hydrocortisone group [80]. Surviving Sepsis campaign does not recommend using routine intravenous hydrocortisone for treatment of adult septic shock patients if adequate fluid resuscitation and vasopressor therapy are able to restore hemodynamic stability [37]. Low dose IV hydrocortisone can be used if patient remains hemodynamicaly unstable despite adequate fluid resuscitation and vasopressor therapy. There is a subset of patients who have relative or absolute adrenal deficiency. The group of adult patients with septic shock with an inappropriately low random cortisol level (< 18 μg/dL) should receive hydrocortisone [81]. Bolus IV hydrocortisone may lead to increase in blood glucose. With continuous infusion, this effect is not detectable [82]. Adverse events with corticosteroid treatment (gastroduodenal bleeding, superinfections, neuromuscular weakness, hyperglycemia and hypernatremia) should be kept in mind [83].

Insulin Therapy: Sepsis induces insulin resistance and hyperglycemia. Corticosteroids are often used for reversal of fluid- and vasopressor-resistant septic shock which aggravates illness-induced hyperglycemia. Both low and high blood glucose values are independently associated with increased mortality [84]. Data have confirmed that hyperglycemia is associated with an increase in death and infection in critically ill patient [85]. Normoglycaemia in Intensive Care Evaluation & Survival Using Glucose Algorithm Regulation (NICE-SUGAR) study data showed intensive insulin therapy significantly increases the risk of hypoglycemia and conferred no overall mortality benefit among critically ill patients [86, 87]. American Association of Clinical Endocrinologists and American Diabetes Association Consensus Statement recommends to initiate Insulin therapy for blood glucose level more than 180 mg/dl (10.0 mmol/l). Once insulin therapy has been started, a glucose range of 140 –180 mg/dl (7.8 –10.0 mmol/l) should be maintained [88]. Intravenous insulin infusions are the preferred method.

Recombinant Activated Protein C: Following the Prospective Recombinant Human Activated Protein C Worldwide Evaluation in Severe Sepsis (PROWESS) trial recombinant human activated protein C was approved for use in adult patients in 2001 [89]. But later studies of recombinant human activated protein C in severe sepsis have shown that it is ineffective in less severely ill patients with severe sepsis as well as in children [90, 91]. The drug was withdrawn from the market and is no longer available following the the latest Prospective Recombinant Human Activated Protein C Worldwide Evaluation in Severe Sepsis and Septic Shock (PROWESS SHOCK) trial which showed that it did not significantly reduce mortality in patients with septic shock [92]. The risk-benefit ratio does not favour its use in sepsis.

Deep Vein Thrombosis Prophylaxis: Most of the septic patients will end up in either ICU or High dependency unit. They are at risk for developing deep vein thrombosis. Patients with severe sepsis should receive daily pharmacoprophylaxis against venous thromboembolism unless heparin use is contraindicated in which case mechanical prophylactic treatment, such as graduated compression stockings or intermittent compression devices are recommended [93]. Daily subcutaneous low-molecular weight heparin has the advantage of lower incidence of heparin-induced thrombocytopenia and is preferred over unfractionated heparin [94].

Specific Treatment of Sepsis Syndrome

The most common sites of infections underlying sepsis are pneumonia, bloodstream infection, intravascular line infection, abdominal infection and urinary tract infection [95, 96, 97, 98]. Skin and soft tissue infections as well as male/female pelvic infections can also lead to sepsis.

Treatment of sepsis syndrome should focus on culture of pertinent sites, early and appropriate pre-emptive antibiotics, aggressive circulatory support, non-injurious ventilator support and prompt infection source control. The spectrum of organisms causing sepsis/ septic shock are changing; In a recent study involving 14,000 ICU patients, Gram negative bacteria were isolated in as many as 62% of patients; Gram positive bacteria in 47% and fungi in 19% of patients [99].

Pre-emptive Antibiotic therapy in sepsis syndrome: Effective pre-emptive antibiotic therapy should be started as soon as the presumptive diagnosis of sepsis syndrome is made. Among hospitalized patients, Kumar et al found that survival was inversely proportional to time to initiation of antibiotics from the onset of septic shock, with an approximately 8%/h absolute decline.

The Surviving Sepsis Campaign, an initiative of the European Society of Intensive Care Medicine, the International Sepsis Forum, and the Society of Critical Care Medicine recommend that intravenous antibiotic therapy should be started within the first hour of recognition of severe sepsis" [37].

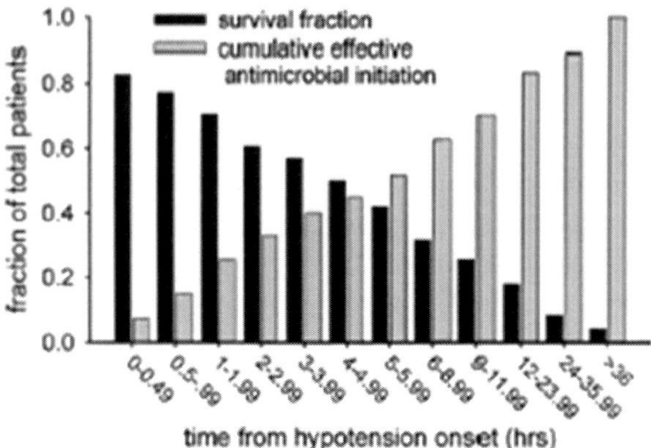

Source: Anand Kumar, Daniel Roberts, Kenneth E. Wood, Bruce Light, Joseph E. Parrillo, Satendra Sharma, Robert Suppes, Daniel Feinstein, Sergio Zanotti, Leo Taiberg, David Gurka, Aseem Kumar, Mary Cheang. Duration of hypotension before initiation of effective antimicrobial therapy is the critical determinant of survival in human septic shock. Crit Care Med 2006; 34:1589–1596.

Figure 4. Cumulative effective antimicrobial initiation following onset of septic shock-associated hypotension and associated survival. The x-axis represents time (hours) following first documentation of septic shock-associated hypotension. Black bars represent the fraction of patients surviving to hospital discharge for effective therapy initiated within the given time interval. The gray bars represent the cumulative fraction of patients having received effective antimicrobials at any given time point.

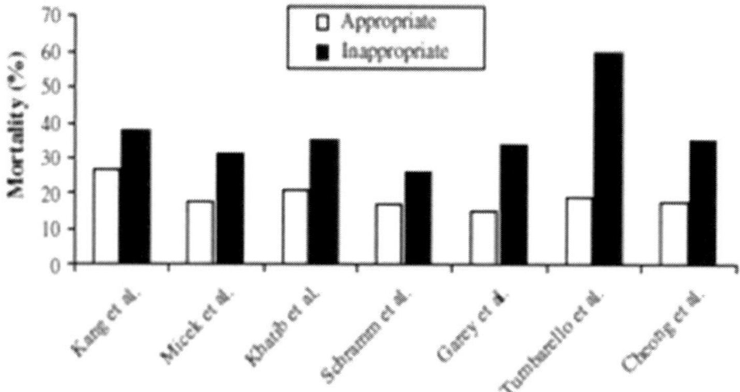

Source: Matthew R. Morrell, Scott T. Micek, Pharm, Marin H. Kollef. The Management of Severe Sepsis and Septic Shock. Infect Dis Clin N Am 23 (2009) 485–501.

Figure 5. Effects of inappropriate and appropriate antimicrobial therapy on mortality in severe sepsis and septic shock.

The most effective agent/agents with an appropriate spectrum based on the site of the infection and a high degree of activity against the presumed pathogens should be used. The concept that site of infection clearly determines organisms should be re-iterated. It has been reported that 23% of patients with sepsis receive inappropriate antibiotic therapy [100]. Based on reports of sepsis outcome, the rates of inappropriate antimicrobial therapy in routine clinical practice may be much higher. Mortality is clearly increased in septic patients who receive inappropriate antibiotic therapy [101, 102].

Patients with severe sepsis/ septic shock warrant sufficiently broad-spectrum antimicrobial coverage against all possible pathogens until the causative organism is identified, at which point, the therapy should be promptly streamlined and de-escalated. The initial selection of antimicrobial therapy should also consider pharmacokinetic profile and provide adequate concentrations at the presumed source of sepsis. Local epidemiologic patterns should be taken into account since the spectrum of activity of most agents remains predictable over short term. Antibiotics given to the patient in the last 3 months should be avoided.

Pneumonia: Pneumonia is the most common cause of Sepsis. Pneumonia may be classified by site of acquisition i.e., hospital/healthcare-acquired pneumonia (HAP) and Community-acquired pneumonia (CAP). Ventilator-associated pneumonia (VAP) is a subset of HAP. From the infectious disease perspective, HAP and VAP are caused by the same pathogens, have the same clinical presentation and require same approach to antimicrobial therapy. There are three HAP and VAP pathogens that have the potential to cause sepsis and septic shock. These are Klebsiella pneumoniae, Staphylococcus aureus and Pseudomonas aeruginosa. Pneumonias caused by these organisms are characterized by high spiking fevers, cyanosis, hypotension and rapid cavitation on chest radiograph [103].

CAPs are not usually associated with severe sepsis or septic shock. However, Klebsiella pneumoniae pneumonia in chronic alcoholics and MSSA/MRSA CAP may present with sepsis and septic shock. Legionella may occasionally cause severe CAP. Viral infections with associated tracheo-bronchial damage predispose to necrotizing hemorrhagic MSSA and MRSA pneumonia with sepsis syndrome and rapid multiorgan system dysfunction.In patients without risk factors for MRSA or Pseudomonas aeruginosa, a potent antipneumococcal beta-lactam plus a macrolide or a respiratory quinolone can be given. In patients with risk factors for Pseudomonas aeruginosa (COPD, frequent previous antimicrobial use, steroid use, bronchiectasis), an antispseudomonal beta-lactum plus an antipseudomonal quinolone may be used initially.

For HAP with severe illness or with suspected multi-drug resistant pathogens, (receipt of antibiotics within the preceding 90 days, current hospitalization of >or = to 5 days, high frequency of antibiotic resistance in the community or in the specific hospital unit, immune suppression or severe septic shock [104]), an anti-pseudomonal beta-lactam, plus an aminoglycoside or an anti-pseudomonal quinolone (depending on local susceptibility data) may be used. MRSA coverage with Vancomycin or Linezolid may be added if MRSA is suspected. Also, if multi- drug resistant Acinetobacter boumanii is suspected, intravenous colistin/Polymixin B may be used. Aerosolised colistin may also be added although data are not conclusive regarding its effectiveness [105]. Based on clinical evaluation at 72 hours and the respiratory secretion gram stain and cultures, antibiotic therapy must be streamlined and de-escalated appropriately.

Blood stream infection: Gram positive sepsis is most commonly caused by staphylococci or enterococci whereas gram-negative sepsis is commonly caused by aerobic gram-negative bacilli, like Escherichia coli and Pseudomonas aeruginosa. Depending on the source, anaerobes and candida species can be a part of the spectrum in polymicrobial infections.

In a study of ICU patients with community-acquired bacteremia, the most common pathogens were Escherechia coli (25%), Steptococcus pneumoniae (16%) and Staphylococcus aureus (14%) [106]. In another study of nursing home patients with bacteremia, the most common pathogens were E.coli (27%), Staphylococcus aureus (18%), and Proteus species (13%) [107]. Hence, if the site of a community acquired infection is not identified, initial antibiotic regimen should target Escherechia coli, Streptococcus pneumoniae and Staphylococcus aureus, including MRSA.Antibiotics with proven efficacy against Staphylococcus aureus like Cloxacillin/ Oxacillin/ Vancomycin/ Daptomycin or Linezolid should be used intravenously. However, Linezolid has not been evaluated sufficiently for bloodstream infections [108, 109, 110, 111]. Other suitable anti-staphylococcal drugs need to be substituted for treatment of isolates with Vancomycin MIC>2mcg/mL [112].

For penicillin susceptible Staphylococcus aureus, crystalline penicillin is the drug of choice [113]. Nafcillin and oxacillin/cloxacillin are the optimal agents for treatment of MSSA bacteremia. Treatment of MSSA bacteremia with Vancomycin is associated with higher mortality and treatment failure, compared to treatment with beta-lactam agents [114, 115]. If Staphylococcal aureus etiology is considered in a severely ill septic patient, a combination of Vancomycin and an anti-staphylococcal penicillin like Nafcillin may be considered, although there are no clinical trials done to prove the benefit of the combination [116].

For gram-negative infections, a beta-lactam agent or a fluoroquinolone may be used depending on the local susceptibility data. In case of penicillin allergic patients, Aztreonam may be safely administered without prior penicillin skin testing. However, an exception is Ceftazidime allergy as they both share a similar side chain. In the SMART study, a global surveillance program, which examined the rates of susceptibility of Enterobacteriaceae isolates from intraabdominal infections to third generation cephalosporins and carbapenems, the ESBL phenotype was found in 28.2% of E.coli isolates and in 22.1% of K. pneumoniae isolates in the Asia-Pacific region. More than half (55.6%) of the E.coli isolates in China were ESBL producers.

In settings with highly antibiotic-resistant pathogens, combination of antibiotics might be relevant. Recent studies have demonstrated that combination therapy including atleast two different classes of antibiotics produces a superior clinical outcome in severely ill patients [117, 118, 119, 120]. Combination therapy might be useful in treatment of neutropenic sepsis and sepsis secondary to Pseudomons aeruginosa. The combination usually consists of a beta lactam agent in combonation with a macrolide/fluoroquinolone/aminoglycoside for select patients. It may also include colistin/ Polymixin B if multi-resistant acinetobacter/ pseudomonas are suspected to be implicated. However, in case of Pseudomonas aeruginosa bacteremia, the association between appropriate antibiotics and improved survival has not been clearly established, perhaps due to importance of host factors [121]. In the setting of a population at low risk of infection with resistant microorganisms, combination therapy has not been found to improve outcomes. When combination therapy is used, it should not be administered for longer than 3-5 days unless clearly needed.

Overwhelming pneumococcal sepsis occurs in patients with asplenia or diminished splenic function. Such patients present with overwhelming sepsis rather than pneumococcal pneumonia even if the initial site of infection is the lungs or upper respiratory tract [122].

Catheter Related Blood stream Infection(CRBSI): CRBSI is predominantly caused by Staphylococci. However, it may be caused by gram negative organisms and fungal pathogens particularly candida species.

Presumptive therapy of CRBSI should include Vancomycin or a potent anti- MRSA agent e.g., Daptomycin. Linezolid is unsuitable for CRBSI. [123] In patients with neutropenia or severe sepsis, empiric gram-negative therapy, including Pseudomonas aeruginosa is appropriate. Patients should be evaluated for the possibility of infection with drug-resistant pathogens and fungal infection. Empirical antifungal therapy should be used in patients at high risk for invasive candidiasis. In severely ill patients, an echinocandin is preferred [124].

Catheter should be removed at the earliest possible. Especially in case of infection with Staphylococcus aureus, enterococci, gram negative bacilli, fungi, and mycobacteria, salvage of the catheter should not be attempted [125].

Abdominal infection: Sepsis related to gastrointestinal tract is caused by fecal flora. Fecal flora is predominantly anaerobic with Bacteroides fragilis predominating (approximately 75%). Most of the remaining fecal flora are common coliforms (approximately 20%) and less common aerobic gram negatives, including P. aeruginosa, especially in patients with recent antibiotic exposure. The rest are enterococci (approximately 5%). Because enterococci are "permissive" pathogens in the gastrointestinal tract (unlike in biliary and urinary tracts), they may not need to be targeted in most cases.

Biliary tract sepsis is usually due to Escherechia coli, Klebsiella pneumoniae, or Enterococcus faecalis. Sepsis syndrome related to liver abscess is caused by same organisms as in the gastrointestinal tract because the portal blood supply is derived from the colon.

Treatment of abdominal infections should involve gram-negative therapy along with coverage against anaerobes. Beta-lactam/beta-lactamase inhibitor combinations, Ciprofloxacin plus metronidazole or Moxifloxacin are suitable candidates. Choice of agent should be based on local antibiotic susceptibility data.

Urinary tract infection: Uropathogens causing urosepsis originate from the gastro-intestinal tract and expectedly are aerobic gram negative organisms or enterococci, usually Enterococcus faecalis. In hospital-acquired urosepsis related to urologic instrument-tation procedures, Pseudomonas aeruginosa is a significant pathogen. Pseudomonas aertuginosa may also be associated with urological obstruction, urolithiasis and chronic prostatitis.

Treatment of Urosepsis should most certainly involve gram-negative therapy. Choice of antibiotic should be based on urine gram stain, local antimicrobial susceptibility patterns and the patient's previous urine culture results, if available. Pseudomonas aeruginosa coverage should be based on the risk factors. An aminoglycoside may be added if resistant organisms are suspected, until cultures are available. Empirical Vancomycin, based on urine gram stain, is reasonable in a severely ill patient.

Skin and soft tissue infection: Sepsis may result from complicated skin and skin-structure infections. Toxic shock syndrome from staphylococcal infections and streptococcal infections with or without necrotizing fasciitis has a disproportionately high rate of morbidity and mortality. Antibiotic therapy should target Gram positive, Gram negative and anaerobic organisms although Group A streptococcus and Clostridium species should be specially considered. Severe necrotising infections of skin and soft tissue should be pre-emptively treated with broad spectrum antibiotics including a beta-lactam/beta-lactamase inhibitor combination or a carbapenem PLUS an anti-staphylococcal agent, preferably with coverage against MRSA. Clindamycin (600 to 900mg q8h intravenous, or Linezolid is recommended to be included in the empiric regimens to treat severe soft tissue infections to enhance killing of organisms in stationary growth and to decrease toxin production [126]. Antibiotic therapy should be tailored based on gram-stain, culture and sensitivity results, once available. Use of high dose IVIG may be beneficial in severe Group A Streptococcal infections [127, 128]. Prompt and early surgical debridement of necrotizing tissue is the mainstay of treatment. Clostridial myonecrosis or Gas gangrene is primarily a toxin-mediated disease, secondary to clostridial exotoxins. The treatment of gas gangrene is primarily surgical to remove devitalized tissue.

Community acquired MRSA (CA-MRSA): CA-MRSA is a newly recognized cause of sepsis and septic shock, related to mainly skin and soft tissue infections, especially infections with strains that are PVL gene positive as they are highly virulent. While CA-MRSA strains may be susceptible to clindamycin, trimethoprim-sulphamethoxazole or doxycycline, it is prudent to treat all MRSA strains with antibiotics that are known to have activity against Health Care associated-MRSA. Therefore, in patients with sepsis or septic shock due to MRSA, it is prudent to use one of the anti-MRSA drugs (i.e., Vancomycin, daptomycin, linezolid) with proven clinical efficacy. Caution should be exercised while treating CA-MRSA with clindamycin as CA-MRSA may exhibit inducible clindamycin resistance during treatment [129].

Female Pelvic Infections: Female pelvic system infections have their microbiologic origin in one of three sources – vaginal microflora, intestinal microflora and sexual transmission [130]. Hence, the usual treatment of female pelvic infection, usually consists of 2nd generation cephalosporin like Cefoxitin and doxycycline. However, there is known the association of female pelvic infections caused by Staphylococcal aureus, Group A Streptococcus and Clostridium sordelli with toxic shock syndrome [131, 132]. These need to be considered in severely ill patients and treated optimally.

Male Pelvic infections: Acute bacterial prostatitis could occasionally lead to severe sepsis. The organisms implicated are predominantly aerobic gram negative organisms, from the GI flora. Burkholderia pseudomallei (Melioid) may be implicated as well in endemic areas in S-E Asia and Northern Australia as a cause of prostatic abscess and sepsis. Also, gram positive cocci like Staphylococcus aureus, enterococcus and streptococci can occasionally cause severe acute bacterial prostatitis, leading to bacteremia and severe sepsis.Treatment should mainly cover gram negative organisms unless the urinary/ prostatic secretion gram stain shows cocci, in which case Nafcillin or Vancomycin may be used, depending on the risk factors for MRSA.

Meningitis: Acute bacterial meningitis is predominantly caused by Streptococcus pneumoniae, in more than 70% of cases followed by Neisseria meningitides. The incidence of Listeria meningitis increases with increasing age.For presumed bacterial meningitis, a combination of Ceftriaxone or Cefotaxime and Vancomycin in meningitis dosages is recommended to cover for the increasing incidence of penicillin resistant pneumococci. In adults over 50 years, ampicillin is added to treat Listeria monocytogenes. Adjunctive dexamethasone for 2-4 days may be added when the etiological agent of meningitis is Streptococcus pneumoniae [133, 134].

Sepsis due to Viral infection: In patients with suspected / confirmed severe Influenza, early antiviral treatment should be initiated with an appropriate antiviral agent.

Source Control

Drainage of closed space infection, removal of infected foreign bodies, and debridement of devitalized tissue are extremely important for source control in sepsis. If intravascular access devices are a possible source of sepsis, they should be promptly removed once an alternate vascular access has been established. Intervention for source control should be undertaken promptly and preferably within the first 24 hours after the diagnosis is made.

Continuation of Antimicrobial Therapy

In general, 7-10 days of antibiotic treatment is adequate unless there are issues with source control. Most documented bacteremias or candidemias are treated for at least 14 days; Staphylococcus aureus bacteremia is generally treated for four weeks because of the high incidence of tissue seeding. However, antibiotics should be continued for a longer time in patients with slow response; in patients with undrainable foci of infection and in patients with immunologic defeciencies. If the source of sepsis is infective endocarditis or other deep seated infections, duration of antibiotic therapy should be targeted toward those. In managing sepsis/septic shock, clinicians should be cognizant that blood cultures may be negative in 50-70% of patients despite being caused by bacteria or fungi [135, 136, 137]. Hence the decision to continue, taper, or stop antibiotic therapy may have to be made on the basis of clinical information alone.

Re-evaluation, particularly by day 3, is important to review culture results and to decide on continuation/ change of antibiotics. Once the patient improves, de-escalation and streamlining of antibiotics should be done. Antibiotic stewardship may reduce the likelihood that the patient will develop super-infection with other organisms like Clostridium difficile, Vancomycin resistant enterococcus or Candida species and this has been shown to be safe [138]. The role of low procalcitonin in discontinuation of empiric antibiotics with probable sepsis, but without culture evidence of infection remains controversial. Cycling of antibiotics has not been shown to decrease development of resistance amongst micro-organisms. Rather, heterogeneity in selection of antibiotics is helpful in decreasing the resistance potential [139].

Every attempt should be made to avoid unnecessarily treating isolates that represent colonization rather than infection. The most common errors made in this regard relate to treating isolates from respiratory secretions in ventilated patients in ICUs and treating colonizing organisms in the urine of patients with indwelling urinary catheters.

Public Health Implications

The burden of sepsis and sepsis survivors is substantial and an under recognized public health problem with major implications for patients, families, and the health care system. Economically, the costs of sepsis are staggering and total tens of billions of dollars annually. Critically ill patients who survive sepsis have an increased risk of recurrent infections, re-admission in the year following their septic episode that is associated with increased mortality [140, 141]. Sepsis is especially common in the elderly and is likely to increase substantially as the population ages. Severe sepsis in older population is independently associated with substantial and persistent new cognitive impairment and functional disability [142]. Trends are showing that, more admissions ends with discharge to a long-term care facility [3].

To summarize, sepsis and septic shock, we wish to end with the following quote:

> "I suspect that the host is caught up in mistaken, inappropriate and unquestionably self-destructive mechanisms by the very multiplicity of defenses available to him, defenses which do not seem to have been designed to operate in net co-ordination with each other. The end result is not defense, it is an agitated, committee-directed, harum-scarum effort to make war."
>
> Lewis Thomas
> The Immunopathology of Inflammation, 1971.

References

[1] Moss M, Martin GS. A global perspective on the epidemiology of sepsis. *Intensive Care Med.* 2004; 30:527–9.

[2] Dombrovskiy VY, Martin AA, Sunderram J, Paz HL. Rapid increase in hospitalization and mortality rates for severe sepsis in the United States: a trend analysis from 1993 to 2003. *Crit. Care Med.* 2007 Vol. 35 No. 5, 1244- 1250.

[3] Gagan Kumar, Nilay Kumar, Amit Taneja, Thomas Kaleekal, Sergey Tarima, Emily McGinley, Edgar Jimenez, Anand Mohan, Rumi Ahmed Khan, Jeff Whittle, Elizabeth Jacobs, Rahul Nanchal. Nationwide Trends of Severe Sepsis in the 21st Century (2000-2007). *Chest.* 2011; 140(5):1223-1231.

[4] Greg S. Martin, David M. Mannino, Marc Moss. The effect of age on the development and outcome of adult sepsis. *Crit. Care Med.* 2006; 34:15–21.

[5] Derek C. Angus, Walter T. Linde-Zwirble, Jeffrey Lidicker, Gilles Clermont. Joseph Carcillo, Michael R. Pinsky. Epidemiology of severe sepsis in the United States: Analysis of incidence, outcome, and associated costs of care. *Crit. Care Med.* 2001; 29:1303–1310.

[6] Martin GS, Mannino DM, Eaton S, et al: The epidemiology of sepsis in the United States from 1979 through 2000. *N. Engl. J. Med.* 2003; 348:1546–1554.

[7] Florian B. Mayr, Sachin Yende, Walter T. Linde-Zwirble, Octavia M. Peck-Palmer, Amber E. Barnato, Lisa A. Weissfeld. Infection Rate and Acute Organ Dysfunction Risk as Explanations for Racial Differences in Severe Sepsis. *JAMA.* 2010;303(24):2495-2503.

[8] Marc Moss. Epidemiology of Sepsis: Race, Sex, and Chronic Alcohol Abuse. *Clinical Infectious Diseases* 2005; 41:S490–7.

[9] Esper AM, Moss M, Martin GS. The effect of diabetes mellitus on organ dysfunction with sepsis: an epidemiologic study. *Crit. Care.* 2009; 13:R18.

[10] Benfield T, Jensen JS, Nordestgaard BG. Influence of diabetes and hyperglycaemia on infectious disease hospitalisation and outcome. *Diabetologia.* 2007;50:549–554.

[11] Prashant Nasa, Deven Juneja, Omender Singh, Rohit Dang, Vikas Arora. Severe Sepsis and its Impact on Outcome in Elderly and Very Elderly Patients Admitted in Intensive Care Unit. *Journal of Intensive Care Medicine*. 2012, 27(3) 179-183.

[12] Jonathan S. Boomer, Kathleen To, Kathy C. Chang, Osamu Takasu, Dale F. Osborne, Andrew H. Walton, Traci L. Bricker, Stephen D. Jarman II, Daniel Kreisel, Alexander S. Krupnick, Anil Srivastava, Paul E. Swanson, Jonathan M. Green, Richard S. Hotchkiss. Immunosuppression in Patients Who Die of Sepsis and Multiple Organ Failure . *JAMA*. 2011;306(23):2594-2605.

[13] Li Ping Chung, Grant W. Waterer. Genetic predisposition to respiratory infection and sepsis., *Critical Reviews in Clinical Laboratory Sciences*, 2011; 48(5-6): 250–268.

[14] Laura J. Moore, Frederick A. Moore, Stephen L. Jones, Jiaqiong Xu, Barbara L. Bass. Sepsis in general surgery: a deadly complication. *The American Journal of Surgery* (2009) 198, 868–874.

[15] Alan C. Heffner, James M. Horton, Michael R. Marchick, Alan E. Jones. Etiology of Illness in Patients with Severe Sepsis Admitted to the Hospital from the Emergency Department. *Clinical Infectious Diseases* 2010; 50:814–820.

[16] Cornbleet PJ. Clinical utility of the band count. *Clin. Lab. Med.* 2002;22(1):101–36.

[17] Wenz B, Gennis P, Canova C, et al. The clinical utility of the leukocyte differential in emergency medicine. *Am. J. Clin. Pathol.* 1986;86(3): 298–303.

[18] Callaham M. Inaccuracy and expense of the leukocyte count in making urgent clinical decisions. *Ann. Emerg. Med.* 1986;15(7):774–81.

[19] Vanderschueren S, De Weerdt A, Malbrain M, et al. Thrombocytopenia and prognosis in intensive care. *Crit. Care Med.* 2000;28(6):1871–6.

[20] Rivers E, Nguyen B, Havstad S, et al. Early goal-directed therapy in the treatment of severe sepsis and septic shock. *N. Engl. J. Med.* 2001;345(19):1368–77.

[21] Gallagher EJ, Rodriguez K, Touger M. Agreement between peripheral venous and arterial lactate levels. *Ann. Emerg. Med.* 1997;29(4):479–83.

[22] Bernard GR, Vincent JL, Laterre PF, et al. Efficacy and safety of recombinant human activated protein C for severe sepsis. *N. Engl. J. Med.* 2001;344(10):699–709.

[23] Kinasewitz GT, Yan SB, Basson B, Universal changes in biomarkers of coagulation and inflammation occur in patients with severe sepsis, regardless of causative micro-organism [ISRCTN74215569]. *Crit. Care* 2004;8(2):R82–90.

[24] Norberg A, Christopher NC, Ramundo ML, et al. Contamination rates of blood cultures obtained by dedicated phlebotomy vs intravenous catheter. *JAMA* 2003; 289:726.

[25] Riedel S, Bourbeau P, Swartz B, et al. Timing of specimen collection for blood cultures from febrile patients with bacteremia. *J. Clin. Microbiol.* 2008; 46:1381.

[26] Päivi Tissari, Alimuddin Zumla, Eveliina Tarkka, Sointu Mero, Laura Savolainen, Martti Vaara, Anne Aittakorpi, Sanna Laakso, Merja Lindfors, Heli Piiparinen, Minna Mäki, Caroline Carder, Jim Huggett, Vanya Gant, Accurate and rapid identification of bacterial species from positive blood cultures with a DNA-based microarray platform: an observational study; *Lancet* 2010; 375: 224–30.

[27] Lee A, Mirrett S, Reller LB, Weinstein MP. Detection of bloodstream infections in adults: how many blood cultures are needed? *J. Clin. Microbiol.* 2007; 45:3546.

[28] Cockerill FR 3rd, Wilson JW, Vetter EA, et al. Optimal testing parameters for blood cultures. *Clin. Infect. Dis.* 2004; 38: 1724.

[29] Patel R, Vetter EA, Harmsen WS, et al. Optimized pathogen detection with 30- compared to 20-milliliter blood culture draws. *J. Clin. Microbiol.* 2011; 49:4047.

[30] Mirrett S, Weinstein MP, Reimer LG, et al. Relevance of the number of positive bottles in determining clinical significance of coagulase-negative staphylococci in blood cultures. *J. Clin. Microbiol.* 2001; 39:3279.

[31] Dahaba AA, Metzler H. Procalcitonin's role in the sepsis cascade. Is procalcitonin a sepsis marker or mediator? *Minerva Anestesiologica* 2009; 75: 447–52.

[32] Shehabi Y, Seppelt I. Pro/con debate: is procalcitonin useful for guiding antibiotic decision making in critically ill patients? *Crit. Care* 2008; 12: 211–6.

[33] Charles PE, Ladoire S, Aho S. et al. Serum procalcitonin elevation in critically ill patients at the onset of bacteremia caused by either Gram-negative or Gram-positive bacteria. *BMC Infect. Dis.* 2008; 8: 38.

[34] Christina Wacker, Anna Prkno, Frank M. Brunkhorst, Peter Schlattmann; Procalcitonin as a diagnostic marker for sepsis: a systematic review and meta-analysis; *Lancet Infect. Dis.* 2013;13: 426–35.

[35] Alvaro Castellanos-Ortega, Borja Suberviola,Luis A. García-Astudillo, María S. Holanda, Fernando Ortiz, Javier Llorca, Miguel Delgado-Rodríguez. Impact of the Surviving Sepsis Campaign protocols on hospital length of stay and mortality in septic shock patients: Results of a three-year follow-up quasi-experimental study. *Crit. Care Med.* 2010; 38:1036 –1043.

[36] Barochia A, Cui X, Vitberg D, et al. Bundled care for septic shock: an analysis of clinical trials. *Crit. Care Med.* 2010; 38:668–678.

[37] R. Phillip Dellinger, Mitchell M. Levy, Andrew Rhodes, Djillali Annane, Herwig Gerlach, Steven M. Opal, Jonathan E. Sevransky, Charles L. Sprung, Ivor S. Douglas, Roman Jaeschke, Tiffany M. Osborn, Mark E. Nunnally, Sean R. Townsend, Konrad Reinhart, Ruth M. Kleinpell, Derek C. Angus, Clifford S. Deutschman, Flavia R. Machado, Gordon D. Rubenfeld, Steven A. Webb, Richard J. Beale, Jean-Louis Vincent, Rui Moreno and the Surviving Sepsis Campaign Guidelines Committee including the Pediatric Subgroup. Surviving Sepsis Campaign: International Guidelines for Management of Severe Sepsis and Septic Shock: 2012 *Crit. Care Med.* 2013; 41:580–637.

[38] Dellinger RP, Levy MM, Carlet JM, et al. Surviving Sepsis Campaign: international guidelines for management of severe sepsis and septic shock. *Intensive Care Med.* 2008;34:17–60.

[39] Dellinger RP, Levy MM, Carlet JM, et al. Surviving Sepsis Campaign: international guidelines for management of severe sepsis and septic shock. *Intensive Care Med.* 2008;34:17–60.

[40] LeDoux D, Astiz ME, Carpati CM, et al. Effects of perfusion pressure on tissue perfusion in septic shock. *Crit. Care med.* 2000;28:2729–32.

[41] A΄lvaro Castellanos-Ortega, Borja Suberviola, Luis A. García-Astudillo, María S. Holanda, Fernando Ortiz, Javier Llorca, Miguel Delgado-Rodríguez. Impact of the Surviving Sepsis Campaign protocols on hospital length of stay and mortality in septic shock patients: Results of a three-year follow-up quasi-experimental study *Crit. Care Med.* 2010;38: 1036-1043.

[42] Perner A, Haase N, Wiis J, White JO, Delaney A. Central venous oxygen saturation for the diagnosis of low cardiac output in septic shock patients. *Acta Anaesthesiol. Scand.* 2009; 54 (1): 98 – 102.

[43] Leone M, Blidi S, Antonini F, et al. Oxygen tissue saturation is lower in nonsurvivors than in survivors after early resuscitation of septic shock. *Anesthesiology* 2009;111(2):366–71.

[44] Mark E. Mikkelsen, Andrea N. Miltiades, David F. Gaieski,Munish Goyal, Barry D. Fuchs,Chirag V. Shah, Scarlett L. Bellamy, Jason D. Christie. Serum lactate is associated with mortality in severe sepsisindependent of organ failure and shock. *Crit. Care Med.* 2009; 37:1670 –1677.

[45] H Bryant Nguyen, Manisha Loomba, James J. Yang, Gordon Jacobsen, Kant Sha, Ronny M Otero, Arturo Suarez, Hemal Parekh, Anja Jaehne, Emanuel P. Rivers. Early lactate clearance is associated with biomarkers of inflammation, coagulation, apoptosis, organ dysfunction and mortality in severe sepsis and septic shock. *Journal of Inflammation* 2010, 7:6.

[46] Emanuel P. Rivers, James A. Kruse, Gordon Jacobsen, Kant Shah, Manisha Loomba, Ronny Otero, Ed W. Childs. The influence of early hemodynamic optimization on biomarker patterns of severe sepsis and septic shock. *Crit. Care Med.* 2007; 35:2016–2024.

[47] Tim C. Jansen, Jasper van Bommel, F. Jeanette Schoonderbeek, Steven J. Sleeswijk Visser, Johan M. van der Klooster, Alex P. Lima, Sten P. Willemsen, Jan Bakker.Early Lactate-Guided Therapy in Intensive Care Unit Patients. *Am. J. Respir. Crit. Care Med.* Vol 182. pp 752–761, 2010.

[48] Michael A. Puskarich, Stephen Trzeciak, Nathan I. Shapiro, Andrew B. Albers, Alan C. Heffner, Jeffrey A. Kline, Alan E. Jones. Whole Blood Lactate Kinetics in Patients Undergoing Quantitative Resuscitation for Severe Sepsis and Septic Shock. *Chest* 2013; 143(6):1548–1553.

[49] Ince C. The microcirculation is the motor of sepsis. *Crit. Care* 2005; 9(Suppl 4):S13–9.

[50] Vincent JL, De Backer D. Microvascular dysfunction as a cause of organ dysfunction in severe sepsis. *Crit. Care* 2005;9(Suppl 4):S9–12.

[51] Durairaj L, Schmidt GA. Fluid therapy in resuscitated sepsis: less is more. *Chest* 2008; 133:252–263.

[52] Wiedemann HP, Wheeler AP, Bernard GR, et al. Comparison of two fluid management strategies in acute lung injury. *N. Engl. J. Med.* 2006; 354:2564– 2575.

[53] Farid Sadaka, Mayrol Juarez, Soophia Naydenov, Jacklyn O'Brien. Fluid Resuscitation in Septic Shock: The Effect of Increasing Fluid Balance on Mortality. *Journal of Intensive Care medicine*. February 27, 2013, doi: 10.1177/0885066613478899.

[54] Fluid resuscitation in septic shock: A positive fluid balance and elevated central venous pressure are associated with increased mortality. John H. Boyd, Jason Forbes, Taka-aki Nakada, Keith R. Walley, James A. Russell, *Crit. Care Med.* 2011; 39:259 –265.

[55] Sheldon Magder. Fluid status and fluid responsiveness. *Current Opinion in Critical Care* 2010,16:289–296.

[56] Michard F, Lopes M, Auler J-O. Pulse pressure variation: beyond the fluid management of patients with shock. *Crit. Care* 2007; 11:131.

[57] Rivers EP, Kruse JA, Jacobsen G, et al. The influence of early hemodynamic optimization on biomarker patterns of severe sepsis and septic shock. *Crit. Care Med.* 2007; 35:2016–2024.

[58] The SAFE Study Investigators. A Comparison of Albumin and Saline for Fluid Resuscitation in the Intensive Care Unit. *N. Engl. J. Med.* 2004;350:2247-56.

[59] Anthony P. Delaney, Arina Dan, John McCaffrey, Simon Finfer. The role of albumin as a resuscitation fluid for patients with sepsis: A systematic review and meta-analysis. *Crit. Care Med.* 2011; 39:386 –391.

[60] Bayer O, Reinhart K, Kohl M, et al. Effects of fluid resuscitation with synthetic colloids or crystalloids alone on shock reversal, fluid balance, and patient outcomes in patients with severe sepsis: a prospective sequential analysis. *Crit. Care Med.* 2012; 40:2543–2551.

[61] Schortgen F, Lacherade JC, Bruneel F, et al: Effects of hydroxyethylstarch and gelatin on renal function in severe sepsis: A multicentre randomised study. *Lancet* 2001; 357:911–916.

[62] Perner A, Haase N, Guttormsen AB, et al; 6S Trial Group; Scandinavian Critical Care Trials Group: Hydroxyethyl starch 130/0.42 versus Ringer's acetate in severe sepsis. *N. Engl. J. Med.* 2012; 367:124–134.

[63] Nicolai Haase and Anders Perner. Hydroxyethyl starch for resuscitation. *Curr. Opin. Crit. Care* 2013, 19:321–325.

[64] Monnet X, Jabot J, Maizel J, et al: Norepinephrine increases cardiac preload and reduces preload dependency assessed by passive leg raising in septic shock patients. *Crit. Care Med.* 2011; 39:689–694.

[65] Sakr Y, Reinhart K, Vincent JL, et al: Does dopamine administration in shock influence outcome? Results of the Sepsis Occurrence in Acutely Ill Patients (SOAP) Study. *Crit. Care Med.* 2006; 34:589–597.

[66] Daniel De Backer, Cesar Aldecoa, Hassane Njimi, Jean-Louis Vincent. Dopamine versus norepinephrine in the treatment of septic shock: A meta-analysis *Crit. Care Med.* 2012; 40:725–730.

[67] Tajender S. Vasu, Rodrigo Cavallazzi, Amyn Hirani, Gary Kaplan, Benjamin Leiby, Paul E. Marik. Norepinephrine or Dopamine for Septic Shock: A Systematic Review of Randomized Clinical Trials. *Journal of Intensive Care Medicine* 27(3) 172-178.

[68] De Backer D, Biston P, Devriendt J, et al. Comparison of dopamine and norepinephrine in the treatment of shock. *N. Engl. J. Med.* 2010; 362(9):779-789.

[69] Sharshar T, Blanchard A, Paillard M, et al: Circulating vasopressin levels in septic shock. *Crit. Care Med.* 2003; 31:1752–1758.

[70] Noguera I, Medina P, Segarra G, et al. Potentiation by vasopressin of adrenergic vasoconstriction in the rat isolated mesenteric artery. *Br. J. Pharmacol.* 1997; 122:431–438.

[71] Dünser MW, Mayr AJ, Ulmer H, et al: Arginine vasopressin in advanced vasodilatory shock: A prospective, randomized, controlled study. *Circulation* 2003; 107:2313–2319.

[72] Morelli A, Ertmer C, Lange M, et al: Effects of short-term simultaneous infusion of dobutamine and terlipressin in patients with septic shock: The DOBUPRESS study. *Br. J. Anaesth.* 2008; 100:494–503.

[73] Broking K, Lange M, Morelli A, et al. Employing dobutamine as a useful agent to reverse the terlipressin-linked impairments in cardiopulmonary hemodynamics and global oxygen transport in healthy and endotoxemic sheep. *Shock* 2008; 29: 71–7.

[74] Anand Kumar, Daniel Roberts, Kenneth E. Wood, Bruce Light, Joseph E. Parrillo, Satendra Sharma, Robert Suppes, Daniel Feinstein, Sergio Zanotti, Leo Taiberg, David Gurka, Aseem Kumar, Mary Cheang. Duration of hypotension before initiation of effective antimicrobial therapy is the critical determinant of survival in human septic shock. *Crit. Care Med.* 2006; 34:1589–1596.

[75] Hang-Cheng Chen, Wen-Ling Lin, Chi-Chun Lin, Wen-Han Hsieh, Cheng-Hsien Hsieh, Meng-Huan Wu, Jiunn-Yih Wu, Chien-Chang Lee. Outcome of inadequate empirical antibiotic therapy in emergency department patients with community-onset bloodstream infections. *J. Antimicrob. Chemother.* 2013; 68: 947–953.

[76] David F. Gaieski, Mark E. Mikkelsen, Roger A. Band, Jesse M. Pines, Richard Massone, Frances F. Furia, Frances S. Shofer, Munish Goyal. Impact of time to antibiotics on survival in patients with severe sepsis or septic shock in whom early goal-directed therapy was initiated in the emergency department. *Crit. Care Med.* 2010; 38:1045–1053.

[77] Djillali Annane, Jean-Marc Cavaillon. Corticosteroids In Sepsis: From Bench To Bedside?. *Shock.* 2003;20(3): 197-207.

[78] Kaufmann I, Briegel J, Schliephake F, et al. Stress doses of hydrocortisone in septic shock: beneficial effects on opsonization-dependent neutrophil functions. *Intensive Care Med.* 2008;34(2):344-349.

[79] Michael Oppert, Ralf Schindler, Claudia Husung, Katrin Offermann, Klaus-Jürgen Gräf, Olaf Boenisch, Detlef Barckow, Ulrich Frei, Kai-Uwe Eckardt. Low-dose hydrocortisone improves shock reversal and reduces cytokine levels in early hyperdynamic septic shock. *Crit. Care Med.* 2005; 33:2457–2464.

[80] Charles L. Sprung, Djillali Annane, Didier Keh, Rui Moreno, Mervyn Singer, Klaus Freivogel, Yoram G. Weiss, Julie Benbenishty, Armin Kalenka, Helmuth Forst, Pierre-Francois Laterre, Konrad Reinhart, Brian H. Cuthbertson, Didier Payen, Josef Briegel. Hydrocortisone Therapy for Patients with Septic Shock. *N. Engl. J. Med.* 2008;358: 111-24.

[81] Djillali Annane, Véronique Sébille, Claire Charpentier, Pierre-Edouard Bollaert, Bruno François, Jean-Michel Korach, Gilles Capellier, Yves Cohen, Elie Azoulay, Gilles Troché, Philippe Chaumet-Riffaut, Eric Bellissant. Effect of Treatment With Low Doses of Hydrocortisone and Fludrocortisone on Mortality in Patients With Septic Shock. *JAMA* 2002; 288:862–871.

[82] Carstens S, Deja M, Bercker S, et al: Impact of bolus application of low-dose hydrocortisone on glycemic control in septic shock patients. *Intensive Care Med.* 2007; 33:730–733.

[83] Djillali Annane, Eric Bellissant, Pierre-Edouard Bollaert, Josef Briegel, Marco Confalonieri, Raffaele De Gaudio, Didier Keh, Yizhak Kupfer, Michael Oppert, G. Umberto Meduri. Corticosteroids in the Treatment of Severe Sepsis and Septic Shock in Adults A Systematic Review. *JAMA*. 2009;301(22):2362-2375.

[84] Sean M. Bagshaw, Moritoki Egi, Carol George, MBus (IT), Rinaldo Bellomo. Early blood glucose control and mortality in critically ill patients in Australia. *Crit. Care Med.* 2009; 37:463– 470.

[85] Mercedes Falciglia, Ron W. Freyberg, Peter L. Almenoff, David A. D'Alessio, Marta L. Render. Hyperglycemia–related mortality in critically ill patients varies with admission diagnosis. *Crit. Care Med.* 2009; 37:3001–3009.

[86] Donald E. G. Griesdale, Russell J. de Souza RD, Rob M. van Dam, Daren K. Heyland, Deborah J. Cook, Atul Malhotra, Rupinder Dhaliwal RD, William R. Henderson, Dean R. Chittock, Simon Finfer, Daniel Talmor. Intensive insulin therapy and mortality among critically ill patients: a meta-analysis including NICE-SUGAR study data. *CMAJ* 2009;180(8):821-827.

[87] The NICE-SUGAR Study Investigators. Intensive versus Conventional Glucose Control in Critically Ill Patients. *N. Engl. J. Med.* 2009;360: 1283-97.

[88] Etie. S. Moghissi, Mary T, Ary Korytkowski, Monica Dinardo, Daniel Einhorn, Richard Hellman, Irl B. Hirsch, Silvio E. Inzucchi, Farmarz Ismail–Belgi, M. Sue Kirkman, Guillermo EUmpierrez. American Association of Clinical Endocrinologists and American Diabetes Association Consensus Statement on Inpatient Glycemic Control. *Diabetes Care* 2009; 32:1119–1131.

[89] PROWESS study group. Eficacy and safety of recombinant human activated protein C for severe sepsis. *N. Engl. J. Med.* 2001;344:699-709.

[90] Administration of Drotrecogin Alfa (Activated) in Early Stage Severe Sepsis (ADDRESS) Study Group. Drotrecogin Alfa (Activated) for Adults with Severe Sepsis and a Low Risk of Death. *N. Engl. J. Med.* 2005;353:1332-41.

[91] Simon Nadel, Brahm Goldstein, Mark D. Williams, Heidi Dalton, Mark Peters, William L. Macias, Shamel A. Abd-Allah, Howard Levy, Robinette Angle, Dazhe Wang, David P. Sundin, Brett Giroir. Drotrecogin alfa (activated) in children with severe sepsis: a multicentre phase III randomised controlled trial. *Lancet* 2007; 369: 836–843.

[92] The PROWESS-SHOCK Study Group. Drotrecogin Alfa (Activated) in Adults with Septic Shock. *N. Engl. J. Med.* 2012;366:2055-64.

[93] Clive Kearon, Elie A. Akl, Anthony J. Comerota, Paolo Prandoni, Henri Bounameaux, Samuel Z. Goldhaber, Michael E. Nelson, Philip S. Wells, Michael K. Gould, Francesco Dentali, Mark Crowther, Susan R. Kahn. Antithrombotic Therapy for VTE Disease. Antithrombotic Therapy and Prevention of Thrombosis, 9th ed: American College of Chest Physicians Evidence-Based Clinical Practice Guidelines. *CHEST* 2012; 141(2)(Suppl):e419S–e494S.

[94] The PROTECT Investigators for the Canadian Critical Care Trials Group and the Australian and New Zealand Intensive Care Society Clinical Trials Group. Dalteparin versus Unfractionated Heparin in Critically Ill Patients. *N. Engl. J. Med.* 2011;364:1305-14.

[95] Angus DC, Linde-Zwirble WT, Lidicker J, Clermont G, Carcillo J, Pinsky MR. Epidemiology of severe sepsis in the United States: analysis of incidence, outcome,and associated costs of care. *Crit. Care Med.* 2001;29:1303-10.

[96] Angus DC, Linde-Zwirble WT, Lidicker J, Clermont G, Carcillo J, Pinsky MR. Epidemiology of severe sepsis in the United States: analysis of incidence, outcome,and associated costs of care. *Crit. Care Med.* 2001;29:1303-10.

[97] Lagu T, Rothberg MB, Shieh MS, Pekow PS, Steingrub JS, Lindenauer PK. Hospitalizations, costs, and outcomes of severe sepsis in the United States 2003 to 2007. *Crit. Care Med.* 2012;40:754-6. [Erratum,Crit Care Med 2012;40:2932.]

[98] Ranieri VM, Thompson BT, Barie PS,et al. Drotrecogin alfa (activated) in adults with septic shock. *N. Engl. J. Med.* 2012; 366:2055-64.

[99] Vincent JL, Rello J, Marshall J, et al. International study of the prevalence and outcomes of infection in intensive care units. *JAMA* 2009;302:2323-9.

[100] Vincent JL, Rello J, Marshall J, et al. International study of the prevalence and outcomes of infection in intensive care units. *JAMA* 2009;302:2323-9.

[101] Harbarth S, Garbino J, Pugin J, Romand JA, Lew D, Pittet D. Inappropriate initial antimicrobial therapy and its effect on survival in a clinical trial of immunomodulating therapy for severe sepsis. *Am. J. Med.* 2003; 115:529–35.

[102] Paul M, Shani V, Muchtar E, Kariv G, Robenshtok E, Leibovici L. Systematic review and meta-analysis of the efficacy of appropriate empiric antibiotic therapy for sepsis. *Antimicrob. Agents Chemother.* 2010;54:4851-63.

[103] Kumar A, Roberts D, Wood KE, et al. Duration of hypotension before initiation of effective antimicrobial the critical determinant of survival in human septic shock. *Crit. Care Med.* 2006;34:1589-94.

[104] Burke A. Cunha, Sepsis and Septic Shock: Selection of Empiric Antimicrobial Therapy, *Crit. Care Clin.* 24(2008) 313-334.

[105] American Thoracic Society, Infectious Diseases Society of America. Guidelines for the management of adults with hospital-acquired, ventilator-associated, and healthcare-associated pneumonia. *Am. J. Respir. Crit. Care Med.* 2005; 171:388.

[106] Kofteridis DP, Alexopoulou C, Valachis A, et al. Aerosolized plus intravenous colistin versus intravenous colistin alone for the treatment of ventilator-associated pneumonia: a matched case-control study. *Clin. Infect. Dis.* 2010; 51:1238.

[107] Valles J, Rello J, Ochagavia A, et al. Community-acquired bloodstream infection in critically ill adult patients: impact of shock and inappropriate antibiotic therapy on survival. *Chest.* 2003;123:1615-1624.

[108] Mylotte JM, Tayara A, Goodnough S. Epidemiology of bloodstream infection in nursing home residents: evaluation in a large cohort from multiple homes. *Clin. Infect. Dis.* 2002;35:1484-1490.

[109] Meka VG, Gold HS. Antimicrobial resistance to linezolid. *Clin. Infect. Dis.* 2004; 39:1010.

[110] Ben Mansour EH, Jacob E, Monchi M, et al. Occurrence of MRSA endocarditis during linezolid treatment. *Eur. J. Clin. Microbiol. Infect. Dis.* 2003; 22:372.

[111] Corne P, Marchandin H, Macia JC, Jonquet O. Treatment failure of methicillin-resistant Staphylococcus aureus endocarditis with linezolid. *Scand. J. Infect. Dis.* 2005; 37:946.

[112] Sánchez García M, De la Torre MA, Morales G, et al. Clinical outbreak of linezolid-resistant Staphylococcus aureus in an intensive care unit. *JAMA* 2010; 303:2260.

[113] Liu C, Bayer A, Cosgrove SE, et al. Clinical practice guidelines by the infectious diseases society of america for the treatment of methicillin-resistant Staphylococcus aureus infections in adults and children. *Clin. Infect. Dis.* 2011; 52:e18.

[114] Nissen JL, Skov R, Knudsen JD, et al. Effectiveness of penicillin, dicloxacillin and cefuroxime for penicillin-susceptible Staphylococcus aureus bacteraemia: a retrospective, propensity-score-adjusted case-control and cohort analysis. *J. Antimicrob. Chemother.* 2013; 68:1894.

[115] Small PM, Chambers HF. Vancomycin for Staphylococcus aureus endocarditis in intravenous drug users. *Antimicrob. Agents Chemother.* 1990; 34:1227.

[116] Chang FY, Peacock JE Jr, Musher DM, et al. Staphylococcus aureus bacteremia: recurrence and the impact of antibiotic treatment in a prospective multicenter study. *Medicine* (Baltimore) 2003; 82:333.

[117] Kevin W. McConeghy, Susan C. Bleasdale, Keith A. Rodvold. The Empirical Combination of Vancomycin and a β-Lactam for Staphylococcal Bacteremia. *Clinical Infectious Diseases* 2013; Advance Access published October 22, 2013, DOI: 10.1093/cid/cit560.

[118] Kumar A, Safdar N, Kethireddy S, et al: A survival benefit of combination antibiotic therapy for serious infections associated with sepsis and septic shock is contingent only on the risk of death: A meta-analytic/ meta-regression study. *Crit. Care Med.* 2010; 38:1651–1664.

[119] Kumar A, Zarychanski R, Light B, et al; Cooperative Antimicrobial Therapy of Septic Shock (CATSS) Database Research Group: Early combination antibiotic therapy yields improved survival compared with monotherapy in septic shock: A propensity-matched analysis. *Crit. Care Med.* 2010; 38:1773–1785.

[120] Micek ST, Welch EC, Khan J, et al: Empiric combination antibiotic therapy is associated with improved outcome against sepsis due to Gram-negative bacteria: A retrospective analysis. *Antimicrob. Agents Chemother.* 2010; 54:1742–1748.

[121] Klastersky J: Management of fever in neutropenic patients with different risks of complications. *Clin. Infect. Dis.* 2004; 39 Suppl 1:S32–S37.

[122] Osih RB, McGregor JC, Rich SE, et al. Impact of empiric antibiotic therapy on outcomes in patients with Pseudomonas aeruginosa bacteremia. *Antimicrob. Agents Chemother.* 2007; 51(13):839–44.

[123] Cunha BA. Ventilator associated pneumonia: Monotherapy is optimal if chosen wisely. *Crit. Care Med.* 2006;10:e141–2.

[124] Pfizer halts pursuit of Zyvox indication based upon mortality signal. *The Pink Sheet* 2007; 69:8.

[125] Clinical practice guidelines for the management of candidiasis: 2009 update by the Infectious Diseases Society of America. Pappas PG, Kauffman CA, Andes D, Benjamin DK Jr, Calandra TF, Edwards JE Jr, Filler SG, Fisher JF, Kullberg BJ, Ostrosky-Zeichner L, Reboli AC, Rex JH, Walsh TJ, Sobel JD, Infectious Diseases Society of America. *Clin. Infect. Dis.* 2009;48(5):503.

[126] Mermel LA, Allon M, Bouza E, et al. Clinical practice guidelines for the diagnosis and management of intravascular catheter-related infection: 2009 Update by the Infectious Diseases Society of America. *Clin. Infect. Dis.* 2009; 49:1.

[127] Streptococcal toxic-shock syndrome: spectrum of disease, pathogenesis, and new concepts in treatment. Stevens DL. *Emerg. Infect. Dis.* 1995; 1(3):69.

[128] Successful management of severe group A streptococcal soft tissue infections using an aggressive medical regimen including intravenous polyspecific immunoglobulin together with a conservative surgical approach. Norrby-Teglund A, Muller MP, Mcgeer A, Gan BS, Guru V, Bohnen J, Thulin P, Low DE. *J. Infect. Dis.* 2005;37(3):166.

[129] Intravenous immunoglobulin G therapy in streptococcal toxic shock syndrome: a European randomized, double-blind, placebo-controlled trial. Darenberg J, Ihendyane

N, Sjölin J, Aufwerber E, Haidl S, Follin P, Andersson J, Norrby-Teglund A, StreptIg Study Group, *Clin. Infect. Dis.* 2003;37(3):333.

[130] Prevalence of inducible clindamycin resistance among community- and hospital-associated Staphylococcus aureus isolates. Patel M, Waites KB, Moser SA, Cloud GA, Hoesley CJ; *Clin. Microbiol.* 2006;44(7):2481.

[131] Faro S. Sepsis in obstetric and gynecologic patients. *Curr. Clin. Topics Infect. Disease* 1999; 19:60-82.

[132] Shands KN, Schmid GP, Dan BB. Toxic-shock syndrome in menstruating women: association with tampon use and Staphylococcus aureus and clinical features in 52 cases. *NEJM* 1980; 303:1436-1442.

[133] Centers for Disease Control. Toxic shock syndrome, United States, 1970-1982. *MMWR.*1982; 31:201.

[134] De Gans J, van de Beek D, European Dexamethasone in Adulthood Bacterial Meningitis Study Investigators. Dexamethasone in adults with bacterial meningitis. *N. Engl. J. Med.* 2002; 347:1549.

[135] Tunkel AR, Hartman BJ, Kaplan SL, et al. Practice guidelines for the management of bacterial meningitis. *Clin. Infect. Dis.* 2004; 39:1267.

[136] Angus DC, Linde-Zwirble WT, Lidicker J, Clermont G, Carcillo J, Pinsky MR. Epidemiology of severe sepsis in the United States: analysis of incidence, outcome, and associated costs of care. *Crit. Care Med.* 2001;29:1303-10.

[137] Abraham E, Reinhart K, Opal S, et al. Efficacy and safety of tifacogin (recombinant tissue factor pathway inhibitor) in severe sepsis: a randomized controlled trial. *JAMA* 2003;290:238-47.

[138] Opal SM, Garber GE, LaRosa SP, et al. Systemic host responses in severe sepsis analyzed by causative microorganism and treatment effects of drotrecogin alfa (activated). *Clin. Infect. Dis.* 2003;37:50-8.

[139] Heenen S, Jacobs F, Vincent JL. Antibiotic strategies in severe nosocomial sepsis: why do we not de-escalate more often? *Crit. Care Med.* 2012;40:1404-9.

[140] Barbosa TM, Levy SB. The impact of antibiotic use on resistance development and persistence. *Drug Resistance Updates* 2000; 3: 303–11.

[141] Sari Karlsson, Esko Ruokonen, Tero Varpula, Tero I. Ala-Kokko, Ville Pettila. Long-term outcome and quality-adjusted life years after severe sepsis. *Crit. Care Med.* 2009; 37: 1268–1274.

[142] Bradford D. Winters, Michael Eberlein, Janice Leung, Dale M. Needham, Peter J. Pronovost, Jonathan E. Sevransky. Long-term mortality and quality of life in sepsis: A systematic review. *Crit. Care Med.* 2010; 38:1276 –1283.

[143] Theodore J. Iwashyna, E. Wesley Ely, Dylan M. Smith, Kenneth M. Langa. Long-term Cognitive Impairment and Functional Disability Among Survivors of Severe Sepsis. *JAMA.* 2010;304(16):1787-1794.

In: Sepsis
Editor: Nancy Khardori

ISBN: 978-1-63117-244-1

Chapter 6

Prevention of Hospital-Acquired Infections in Adults: Focus on "Surviving Sepsis Campaign"

Vidya Sundareshan M.D.*[1], *Rajagopal Sreedhar*[2] *M.D.* and *Nancy Khardori*[3] *M.D., Ph.D.

[1]Division of Infectious Diseases, Department of Internal Medicine, Southern Illinois University School of Medicine, Springfield, Illinois, US

[2]Division of Pulmonary and Critical Care Medicine, Department of Internal Medicine, Southern Illinois University School of Medicine, Springfield, Illinois, US

[3]Division of Infectious Diseases, Department of Internal Medicine and Department of Microbiology and Molecular Cell Biology, Eastern Virginia Medical School, Norfolk, Virginia, US

Abstract

Prevention of hospital acquired infections should be an important goal in all healthcare settings. It becomes even more prudent in the case of patients with sepsis because of heightened morbidity as well as mortality. This chapter explores prevention of hospital acquired infections in adults focusing on surviving sepsis campaign. With the increasing awareness that many of the infections are preventable, the infection control standards nation-wide are becoming higher, particularly in settings such as the Intensive care units (ICU). With improved education, surveillance, infection control practices for prevention as well as early diagnosis, risk for hospital acquired infections in septic patients can be minimized. When infections are identified, prompt treatment with targeted antibiotic therapy and appropriate infection control measures can decrease development of resistance in pathogens. Multi-drug resistance is an emerging problem which should particularly be controlled optimally in the Intensive care units. Lastly, prevention of health care infections is every health care worker's responsibility. Empowering all the staff involved in patient care by educating them about existing guidelines will lead to better outcomes for the patient and decrease health care cost.

Introduction

Hospital acquired infections are infections in a hospitalized patient that were neither present nor incubating at hospital admission. Prevention of hospital acquired infections should be an important goal in all healthcare settings. It becomes even more critical in patients with sepsis because of the heightened morbidity as well as mortality. This chapter explores prevention of hospital acquired infections in adults with a focus on surviving sepsis campaign.

It has been shown that Intensive care units (ICUs) account for fewer than 10 percent of total beds in most hospitals, but more than 20 percent of all nosocomial infections are acquired here [1]. In an International study, 60 percent of the patients in the ICU were noted to be infected [2]. Not only is the incidence of infections higher, the outcomes are also poor. Independently, infection increases the odds of mortality by 1.5 times [2]. The short term and long term outcomes of sepsis compared with hospitalization for causes other than sepsis are outlined in Table 1, which is adapted from Center for Disease Control (CDC)/ National Center for Health Statistics (NCHS), National Hospital Discharge Survey, 2008 [3].

Table 1. Disposition and outcomes in Sepsis as compared with hospitalizations for other diagnoses, 2008

Characteristic	Septicemia or sepsis	Other diagnoses
Disposition	Percent	
Home[1]	39	79
Transfer to other short-term facility[1]	6	3
Transfer to long-term care institution[1]	30	10
Died during the hospitalization[1]	17	2
Other or not stated	8	6
Total	100	100

[1]Difference was noted to be statistically significant.

From the table, it can be seen that there is significant long term morbidity as well as higher mortality in patients with sepsis. From the above, In-hospital deaths were more than eight times as likely in septic patients (17%) compared with patients admitted to the hospital with other diagnoses (2%). Those who survive severe sepsis are more likely to have permanent organ damage [4], cognitive impairment, and physical disability [5]. Patients admitted with a diagnosis of sepsis were only one-half as likely to be discharged home. They were twice as likely to be transferred to other short-term care facilities and three times as likely to be discharged to long-term care institutions as compared with patients admitted for other diagnoses [3].

Surviving sepsis guidelines became available in 2008 and these were endorsed by Infectious diseases Society of America in 2012. Initial resuscitation, screening for sepsis with emphasis on accuracy in diagnosis, anti-microbial therapy, source control, infection prevention, hemodynamics and adjunctive therapy as well as vasopressor, inotropic use, corticosteroid use where applicable, supportive care including mechanical ventilation for sepsis- induced Acute respiratory Distress Syndrome (ARDS), proper use of sedation, analgesia and neuromuscular blockade, optimal blood glucose management, renal replacement therapy with electrolyte replacement, deep venous thrombosis prevention, stress ulcer management and nutrition to meet caloric requirements are all components of the surviving sepsis campaign [6].

Preventive measures for nosocomial infections in these extremely vulnerable patients are one of the essential steps towards working for improved outcomes in patients with Sepsis. It has been shown that infections with susceptible as well as resistant pathogens are higher in patients in the ICU, the risk corresponds to the length of stay in the ICU [7, 8] This could be explained by a higher incidence of chronic comorbid illnesses in these patients compared with other hospitalized patients. Secondly, patients with a diagnosis of sepsis already have abnormalities in cellular, cytokine and coagulation mechanisms contributing to a higher propensity for nosocomial infections [8].Thirdly, these patients have a high frequency of invasive devices (e.g., mechanical ventilators, urinary catheters, or central venous catheters that directly provide a source of entry for microorganisms that may be colonizing or infecting the patients further adding to the burden of nosocomial infections in the ICU [9].

There is more frequent contact with healthcare personnel caring for critically ill patients, which can be another risk factor for hospital acquired infections. The devices and equipment in the ICU setting in itself can be reservoirs of infection even with proper maintenance leading to transmission [9]. Furthermore, high prevalence of nosocomial super infections in critically ill ICU patients can be associated with high antibiotic consumption. With increased antibiotic usage, there is constant pressure for selection and induction of antibiotic resistance [10, 11].

Multidrug-resistant and pan drug resistant pathogens, such as methicillin-resistant Staphylococcus aureus (MRSA), vancomycin-resistant enterococci (VRE), carbapenem-resistant Acinetobacter baumannii, Extended-spectrum beta-lactamases and carbapenemases producing enterobacteriacae, carbapenem-resistant Pseudomonas aeruginosa, are all highly prevalent in the ICU [12-16].

With many states having enacted legislation requiring mandatory public reporting of Health care associated infections, following which, the surveillance has improved nationally. Over 12,000 hospitals, in all 50 states use CDC's National Healthcare Safety Network (NHSN) which is the most widely used healthcare-associated infection tracking system in the United States. To date, 30 states and the District of Columbia require reporting of Health care associated infections using CDC's NHSN.

Although the numbers of nosocomial infections reported in 2011 were considerably higher due to a larger number of hospitals reporting Hospital acquired infections, it allows us to accurately understand the enormity of the problem. Moreover, NHSN provides important surveillance data for facilities, states, regions, and the nation to help identify problem areas, measure progress of prevention efforts, and thereby eliminate healthcare-associated infections [17, 18].

The sections below will discuss the various Hospital acquired Infections particularly in patients presenting with critical illness and the existing guidelines in place for prevention of these infections.

Central Line Associated Blood Stream Infections

According to CDC's 'Guidelines for the Prevention of Intravascular Catheter-Related Infections', published in 2011, there were 15 million catheter related patient days in the ICU during a specific duration in the selected population [19]. In the United States, Central line associated Blood Stream Infections (CLABSI) decreased from 3.64 to 1.65 infections per 1000 central line days between 2001 and 2009 [20]. This amounted to approximately 18,000 central line-related infections in 2009. From the Surveillance and Control of Pathogens of Epidemiologic Importance (SCOPE) database, in 49 hospitals between 1995 and 2002 approximately 51 percent of the total number of CLABSI occurred in the ICU in 49 hospitals [21]. It has been estimated that about 50,000 to 100000 CLABSIs occur per year [19] and it has been estimated that up to 80000 CLABSI can occur in the ICU [19], of a of the total 250,000 Blood Stream Infections (BSI-primary and Secondary infections) occurring hospital-wide [22]. Primary BSI are from Intravascular catheters, mainly central venous catheters and secondary BSI are from other sites such as the urinary tract, skin or lung There are also billions of healthcare dollars spent on line related infections and the associated increased length of stay [23]. One study estimates a marginal cost of $25,000 to the health-care system per episode [24]. The attributable mortality from CLABSIs is estimated to be 12-25% [24]. The attributable mortality for these BSIs has ranged from no increase in mortality in studies that controlled for severity of illness [25-27] to 35% increase in mortality in prospective studies that did not use this control [28, 29]. Infectious Diseases Society of America (IDSA) has endorsed the following guidelines recommended by a multi-specialty working group for health care providers with the goal to prevent CLABSIs from all patient-care areas:

1. Prior to insertion of the central venous catheters, ensure proper education and training of the health care personnel involved in the insertion, care, and maintenance of central venous catheters about CLABSI prevention, indications for use as well as proper procedures for insertion and maintenance of the intravenous catheters (A-II) [30-34, 19, 24]. Please refer to Table 2 in the appendix on the strength of recommendation and quality of evidence. Follow this with periodic assessments of knowledge and adherence to guidelines for all personnel involved in the insertion and maintenance of intravascular catheters. Ensure appropriate nursing staff levels in the ICU. Studies have shown that a high level of pool nurses or high patient to nurse ratio can increase the rate of CLABSI [35, 36].
2. Appropriate selection of the type of catheter and site are important. Recommendations include use of an upper extremity site in adults for catheter insertion. It is recommended to replace a catheter inserted in a lower extremity site to an upper extremity site as soon as possible. (II) The site of catheter insertion can predict the risk for catheter-related infection from the density of local skin flora, phlebitis and risk for thrombophlebitis. For adults, lower extremity insertion sites are associated with a higher risk for infection than are upper extremity sites [37-39]. Although no clinical trials have been done, catheters inserted into an internal jugular vein have been associated with higher risk for infection than those inserted into a subclavian or femoral vein [40-43]. Femoral catheters should be avoided, when possible, because they are associated with a higher risk for deep venous thrombosis

than internal jugular catheters as well as a higher risk of infections due to high rates of colonization. In pediatric patients, upper or lower extremities or the scalp (in neonates or young infants) can be used as catheter insertion site (II) [43, 44]. Selection of catheters must be done on the basis of the intended purpose and duration of use, known infectious and non-infectious complications and experience of the personnel managing the catheter [44]. Polyurethane catheters have been associated with fewer infectious complications than catheters made of polyvinyl chloride or polyethylene [45, 46]. Steel needles have the same rate of infectious complications as do these catheters [44, 46] but can be complicated by infiltration of intravenous (IV) fluids into the subcutaneous tissues. (IA)

3. Follow all recommended central line insertion practices to prevent infection.
4. Hand hygiene and proper aseptic techniques. Hand washing can be with traditional soap and water or alcohol based hand rubs. These should be performed before and after Central venous Catheters (CVC) placements. Avoid palpating the area around the insertion site to maintain asepsis.
5. Maximal Sterile barrier protection with cap, mask, sterile gown, and sterile gloves as well as a sterile body drape for insertion of CVCs including Peripherally Inserted Central Catheters (PICC) and guide wire exchanges. Sterile sleeve to protect pulmonary artery catheter insertions.
6. Adequate skin preparation with an antiseptic before insertion of vascular catheter. chlorhexidine solution > 0.5% with alcohol is preferred. If there is a contraindication for use of chlorhexidine, povidone-iodine, tincture of iodine or 70% alcohol may be used [47, 48]. Catheter site dressing recommendations include use of sterile gauze. There is a recommendation against the use of antibiotics ointments locally at the insertion site as this can promote fungal infections and antimicrobial resistance [49, 50]. Patient cleansing with 2% chlorhexidine washes for daily skin cleaning to reduce CLABSIs. [51-53]
7. Suture less catheter securement devices are recommended to reduce line infections. [54]
8. Use of chlorhexidine/ silversulfa diazine or minocycline/rifampin impregnated CVCs in patients whose catheter is expected to remain in place for >5 days, if rate of CLABSI is still high after implementing the comprehensive strategies of educating staff, use of maximal barrier methods and use of >0.5% chlorhexidine preparation with alcohol for skin antisepsis during CVC insertion. [55-62] The use of minocycline-rifampin seems to have the greatest reduction when compared with other antibiotic impregnated CVCs. (grade 1B) [79]
9. Systemic antibiotics prophylaxis is not recommended prior to CVC insertion. [63] Antibiotic locks, catheter flushes with antibiotics and catheter lock prophylaxis can be used in patients with long term catheters who have multiple CLABSIs despite asepsis in technique of insertion and maintenance.
10. Anticoagulant use through the CVC should be avoided in general population. [64]
11. Recommendation is to avoid replacing peripheral and midline catheters more frequently than 72-96h. Do not routinely replace PICC lines, hemodialysis lines. Avoid guidewire exchanges for non-tunnelled catheter to prevent infection or when suspected to be infected. Avoid removing CVCs or PICCs for fever alone. [65-78]
12. Remove and do not replace umbilical catheters with signs of CLABSI. [80]

13 Fluids infused with lipid emulsions or blood products can enhance microbial growth and therefore require more frequent changes of administration sets. [81-86]

Focusing on surviving sepsis recommendations, the implementation of a central line care bundle, including staff education, creation of a catheter insertion cart, implementation of a checklist to ensure adherence to evidence-based guidelines, empowering nurses to stop catheter insertion procedures when a guideline violation is observed, and daily assessment of possible catheter removal (1B) have all shown to be very effective strategies. Replacement of administration sets every 96 hours (IIA) has also been recommended in surviving sepsis guidelines, except when used for the administration of blood, blood products, or lipids, in which case sets must be changed within 24 hours (1A).

Ventilator-Associated Pneumonias

Ventilator-associated pneumonia (VAP) is defined as the infection of lung tissue in mechanically ventilated patients that develops 48 hours or more after intubation. Hospital Acquired Pneumonia (HAP) is defined as pneumonia that occurs 48 hours or more after admission, which was not incubating at the time of admission [87]. HAP may be managed in a hospital ward or in the intensive care unit (ICU) when the illness is more severe. Health Care Associated Pneumonia (HCAP) includes any patient who was hospitalized in an acute care hospital for two or more days within 90 days of the infection; resided in a nursing home or long-term care facility; received recent intravenous antibiotic therapy, chemotherapy, or wound care within the past 30 days of the current infection; or attended a hospital or hemodialysis clinic [87].

Hospital acquired pneumonia is the second most common hospital-acquired infection and occurs commonly in patients with endotracheal intubation and mechanical ventilation [88]. The development of pneumonia in intubated patients can affect almost 50% of the patients. [90-92] VAP is associated with a higher mortality rate and significantly longer ICU length of stay and hospital costs. [89]

With practices such as education strategies [93, 94] and ventilator bundles [95, 96], VAP can be prevented. Strategies to prevent VAP should be considered in all patients with severe sepsis requiring intubation. [97]

1. Elevation of the head end of the bed to 30 to 45 degrees for all critically ill and mechanically ventilated patients (grade 1B). When unable to elevate head end up to 30 degrees, back-rest elevation of at least 10 degrees should be maintained. Aspiration of upper airway secretions is a common event even in normal healthy adults [98]. Semi recumbent position decreases the incidence of VAP in mechanically ventilated patients as compared with the supine position. [98-100] In patients receiving enteral nutrition, elevation of the head-of-bed elevation is especially effective in reducing the risk of VAP. [98] However, the feasibility of maintaining head-of-bed elevation in daily practice has been questioned by some authors [101, 102]. Some studies were able to considerably decrease infections even with an average head-of-bed elevation of 28 degrees although the target was 45 degrees.

2. Use of an endotracheal tube with subglottic secretion drainage in patients expected to require mechanical ventilation for >72 hours (grade 1A). Impaired gag reflex causes pooling of secretions in the posterior oropharynx [104], and micro aspiration of subglottic secretions leads to VAP. Drainage of Subglottic secretion is facilitated by use of a specially designed endotracheal or tracheotomy tube with a separate dorsal lumen opening above the endotracheal tube cuff. Drainage of Subglottic secretions can effectively prevent VAP in patients expected to be mechanically ventilated for >72 hours (relative risk is estimated at 0.51; 95 % confidence interval 0.37–0.71) [105].
3. Recommendation for using a silver-coated endotracheal tube. (Grade 2A). In multicenter, randomized, controlled trials, a silver-coated endotracheal tube demonstrated to reduce bacterial airway colonization as well as VAP in patients intubated 24 hours or more. [106, 107]
4. Recommendation for using endotracheal tube with a polyurethane cuff (grade 2B). In a single-center, randomized, controlled trial, an endotracheal tube with a polyurethane cuff was shown to significantly reduce early-onset postoperative pneumonia in cardiosurgical patients [108].
5. Endotracheal cuff pressure should be maintained at least 20 cm H_2O, but not >30 cm H_2O (grade 1C). Inadequate cuff pressure is a risk factor for micro aspiration of oropharyngeal secretions and subsequent pneumonia. One observational study among intubated patients not receiving antibiotic therapy showed that a persistent intracuff pressure <20 cm H_2O was an independent predictor of VAP (relative risk, 4.2) [109]. Cuff pressure maintained at the lowest pressure of >20 cm H_2O prevents cuff leak.
6. Heat and moisture exchangers should be changed every 5 to 7 days, or as clinically indicated (grade 2C). Humidification of inspired air to prevent mucosal injury may be achieved by using a heated humidifier, a heated humidifier with a heated wire circuit, or passively using a heat and moisture exchanger. There are insufficient data to demonstrate a benefit in VAP reduction for any humidification device [110]. No benefit in infection rates or functionality of ventilator circuits has been demonstrated when heat and moisture exchangers are changed every day compared to every 5 to 7 days. [111, 112]
7. Ventilator circuits should not be changed routinely, except between patients (grade 1B). There is no evidence that routine ventilator circuit changes can reduce the incidence of VAP [90, 113]. New ventilator circuits should be used for each patient, and circuit changes should be performed only if the circuit becomes visibly soiled or damaged [97].
8. Aspiration of endotracheal secretions in response to clinical signs, i.e., visible or audible signs of respiratory secretions, respiratory deterioration, or other changes in the patient's condition that may be attributable to respiratory secretions in intubated patients (grade 1C). Critically ill patients mechanically ventilated via a tracheal tube frequently require removal of tracheobronchial and upper airway secretions because of increased mucus production and a decreased ability to clear secretions. [114, 115] Secretion removal may reduce infectious, respiratory, and complicate maintenance of tube patency [116-118] Suctioning should only be performed when necessary, using the lowest possible suction pressure, for no longer than 15 seconds, and use

continuous rather than intermittent suctioning; The suction catheter should occlude less than half the lumen of the endotracheal tube and be inserted no further than the carina. Hyper oxygenation should be provided before and after suctioning; and saline lavage should be avoided [116, 117]. The optimum frequency of endotracheal suctioning has not been clearly determined but should be in response to clinical signs. There is insufficient evidence to recommend the benefits of either an open or closed suctioning system [116, 117]

9. Regular mouth care and oral cavity assessment provided to all critically ill and intubated patients (grade 1C). Colonization of the oropharynx by pathogens is a potential risk factor for the development of VAP. [118-123]. Critical illness contributes to changes in the oral flora, and an increase in Gram-negative flora that includes more virulent organisms may occur [124, 125]. Providing regular oral care, incorporating oral cavity assessment, is an important part of providing comfort to the critically ill patient [126] and is also demonstrated to contribute to a decrease in VAP [126-129]. Assessment should include the condition of the teeth, gums, tongue, mucus membranes, and lips, and barriers to mouth care delivery [125]. The use of a designated oral care protocol, in association with an education program for nurses, can increase compliance and assessment of mouth care [131].

Recommendation for the use of chlohexidine-based antiseptic for oral care in intubated patients (grade 1A) [132-135] Chlorhexidine decontaminates the oropharynx [136, 137] and its use in oral care has been proven to decrease dental plaque [138] incidence of respiratory infections, [138] and to substantially decrease the incidence of VAP [140-143] The optimal concentration of chlorhexidine solution for oral care (0.12%, 0.2%, or 2%) remains undetermined. The optimum frequency for oral care with chlorhexidine has not been demonstrated. In general, a frequency of three to four times daily is proposed [132, 143, 144] The use of tooth brushing in critically ill patients as a component of oral care protocols has demonstrated efficacy [128, 129] Tap water should not be used for oral care in the critically ill. [126] IN recent studies and it has been noted that potentially pathogenic bacteria are present in the water supply of health care facilities. Therefore, tap water can be a source of infections. Sterile water may be used of sterile water as a substitute. Currently however, Tap water is used in many critical care units when providing oral care.

The surviving sepsis guidelines, for Infection prevention, stress on selective oral decontamination (SOD) and selective digestive decontamination (grade 2B) as methods that could reduce the incidence of Ventilator associated pneumonia. With oral chlorhexidine gluconate as a form of oropharyngeal decontamination the risk of ventilator-associated pneumonia in ICU patients with severe sepsis can be reduced (grade 1A)

Infectious diseases society of America guidelines for prevention of VAP and health care associated Pneumonias (HCAP)and for reduction in VAP and HCAP with multidrug resistant organisms (MDR) include the following [87]

- A lower respiratory tract culture should to be collected from all patients before antibiotic therapy, but collection of cultures should not delay the initiation of therapy in critically ill patients.
- Either “semiquantitative” or “quantitative” culture data can be used for the management of patients with HAP.

- Lower respiratory tract cultures can be obtained bronchoscopically or nonbronchoscopically, and can be cultured quantitatively or semiquantitatively.
- Quantitative cultures increase specificity of the diagnosis of HAP without deleterious consequences, and the specific quantitative technique should be chosen on the basis of local expertise and experience.
- Negative lower respiratory tract cultures can be used to stop antibiotic therapy in a patient who has had cultures obtained in the absence of an antibiotic change in the past 72 hours.
- Early, appropriate, broad-spectrum, antibiotic therapy should be prescribed with adequate doses to optimize antimicrobial efficacy.
- An empiric therapy regimen should include agents that are from a different antibiotic class than the patient has recently received.
- Combination therapy for a specific pathogen should be used judiciously in the therapy of HAP, and consideration should be given to short-duration (5 days) aminoglycoside therapy, when used in combination with a Beta -lactam to treat P. aeruginosa pneumonia.
- Colistin should be considered as therapy for patients with VAP due to a carbapenem-resistant Acinetobacter species.
- Aerosolized antibiotics may have value as adjunctive therapy in patients with VAP due to some MDR pathogens.
- De-escalation of antibiotics should be considered once data are available on the results of lower respiratory tract cultures and the patient's clinical response.
- A shorter duration of antibiotic therapy (7 to 8 days) is recommended for patients with uncomplicated HAP, VAP, or HCAP who have received initially appropriate therapy and have had a good clinical response, with no evidence of infection with nonfermenting gram-negative bacilli.
- If P. aeruginosa pneumonia is documented, combination therapy is recommended. The principal justification is the high frequency of development of resistance on monotherapy [145]. Although combination therapy will not necessarily prevent the development of resistance, combination therapy is more likely to avoid inappropriate and ineffective treatment of patients (Level II) [146].
- If Acinetobacter species are documented to be present, the most active agents are the carbapenems, sulbactam,colistin, and polymyxin. There are no data documenting an improved outcome if these organisms are treated with a combination regimen (Level II) [147, 148].
- If ESBL producing Enterobacteriaceae are isolated, monotherapy with a third-generation cephalosporin should be avoided. The most active agents are the carbapenems (Level II) [149].
- Adjunctive therapy with an inhaled aminoglycoside or polymyxin for MDR gram-negative pneumonia should be considered, especially in patients who are not improving with systemic therapy alone (Level III) [150].
- Linezolid is an alternative to vancomycin for the treatment of MRSA VAP and may be preferred on the basis of a subset analysis of two prospective randomized trials (Level II) [151-153]. This agent may also be preferred if patients have renal insufficiency or are receiving other nephrotoxic agents, but more data are needed (Level III).

- Antibiotic restriction can limit epidemics of infection with specific resistant pathogens. Heterogeneity of antibiotic prescriptions, including formal antibiotic cycling, may be able to reduce the overall frequency of antibiotic resistance. However, the long-term impact of this practice is unknown. (Level II) [154, 155]

Catheter Associated Urinary Tract Infection (CAUTI)

The burden of disease from CAUTI is significant. Urinary tract infection is the most common hospital-acquired infection; 80% of these infections are due to presence of an indwelling urethral catheter [156, 158]. Twelve to sixteen percent of hospitalized patients receive placement of a urinary catheter at some time during their hospital stay [157]. Bacteremia and sepsis may occur in percentage of these infected patients. [159, 160] The daily risk of acquisition of urinary infection varies from 3% to 7% when an indwelling urethral catheter remains in situ. With 30 million indwelling bladder catheters placed annually nationwide, a large number of patients face an increased risk of developing catheter-associated bacteriuria. Most previous studies assessing morbidity and mortality associated with catheter use have not separated urinary tract infection from asymptomatic bacteriuria.

This has made it difficult to determine if bacteria in the urine puts patients at higher risk for bloodstream infection or death. In a retrospective cohort study of 444 urine cultures from 308 patients, researchers at Baylor College of Medicine found that catheter-associated urinary tract infection, but not asymptomatic bacteriuria, was significantly associated with developing bacteremia within 30 days but was not significantly associated with increased mortality. Treatment with antibiotics did not reduce the risk of developing bacteremia or change mortality rates. [158] Overall mortality is high (21.1 percent), indicating, as expected, that hospitalized patients who require indwelling bladder catheters have many serious underlying illnesses. [158] In 2008, IDSA endorsed the guidelines for prevention of Catheter associated Urinary Tract Infections. [158] Recommendations to prevent CAUTI include:

1 All attempts should be made to limit the duration of urinary catheterization (grade 1C). The urinary tract is the most prevalent source of nosocomial infection and there are several recommendations to prevent or reduce the incidence of UTI. [161] Duration of catheterization is the most important risk factor for development of UTI [161]. Postoperative urinary catheterization >2 days is associated with an increased likelihood of UTI and 30-day mortality, as well as a decreased likelihood of discharge to home [162]. Nurses should advocate for prompt removal of urinary catheters [163] and discourage long-term catheterization, if possible.

2 A sterile, continuously closed drainage system be maintained (grade 1A). Closed urinary drainage systems are pivotal in preventing UTI [163]. The risk of infection reduces from 97% using open systems to 8% to 15% when sterile closed systems are used. [164-166] Errors in maintaining sterile closed drainage and opening the closed drainage system have been well-documented to predispose patients to infection. [164, 166-169]

3 Regular perineal hygiene measures (grade 1C). Most episodes of UTI are caused by the patient's own flora [161]. Daily cleansing of the urethral meatus using soap and water or perineal cleanser is recommended. [163, 170]
4 Maintain unobstructed urine flow (grade 2C). Reflux of urine is associated with infection; therefore, drainage bags should be positioned below the level of the bladder at all times to prevent urine back-flow and unobstructed urine flow should be maintained. [171-173]

Surgical Site Infections

The Centers for Disease Control and Prevention's National Nosocomial Infections Surveillance System [14] and the National Healthcare Safety Network have the following widely used definitions for Surgical Site Infections (SSI). [14, 15]

These Infections that develop 24 to 48 hour after surgery are classified as:

1 Superficial incisional Infections that involve only skin or subcutaneous tissue of the incision
2 Deep Incisional Infections: that involve fascia and muscular layers
3 Organ/Space Infections

The burden of SSI as complication in acute care facilities is high. It occurs in 2%-5% of patients undergoing inpatient surgery in the United States, [174, 175] amounting to approximately 500,000 SSIs each year [174] This results in each SSI to be associated with approximately 7-10 additional postoperative hospital days. [174] Apart from morbidity, it also results 2-11 times higher risk of death, compared with operative patients without an SSI. [176, 177] Seventy-seven percent of deaths in patients with SSI are directly attributable to SSI with an annual health care cost of 4 10 billion. [178]

In 2003, the Surgical Infection Prevention Guidelines became available for antimicrobial prophylaxis in surgery. [106] They recommended that infusion of the first antimicrobial dose should begin within 60 minutes of incision, and when a fluoroquinolone or vancomycin is indicated the infusion should begin within 120 minutes of incision to prevent antibiotic-associated reactions [179, 180]

Perioperative hair removal is associated with increased in skin and soft tissue infections (SSI). It has been shown that the methodology of hair removal such as depilatory cream, razors, clippers compared with no hair removal showed no difference in Skin and Soft Tissue Infection rates among patients who had hair removal before surgery [181-185] However, shaving was associated with significantly more SSIs compared with clipping or depilatory cream [185] Although depilatory creams were associated with a lower SSI risk than shaving or clipping [178] they could produce hypersensitivity reactions [186]. The increased infection risk associated with clipping or shaving is thought to be due to the formation of microscopic cuts in the skin that later act as nidus for bacterial infections [181].

Increased glucose levels (>200 mg/dL) in the immediate postoperative period (≤48 hours) are noted with increased SSI risk [187, 188] Patients with a blood glucose level >300 mg/dL within 48 hours of surgery had more than three-times the likelihood of having wound infections compared to people with controlled blood sugar. [189] Education of nurses regarding frequent monitoring of glucose levels along with timely administration of insulin and hypoglycemic agents can optimize glucose control in patients thereby preventing SSI. Lastly, concurrent remote site infections can increase the risk of post-operative SSI [190-193]. It is recommended that in elective surgeries all infections remote to the surgical site should be treated aggressively.[181]

Infectious Diseases Society of America and Society of healthcare epidemiology of America (SHEA) practice guidelines for surgical site infections includes:

1 Antimicrobial prophylaxis must be administered within 1 hour of incision to maximize tissue concentration. Two hours are allowed for the administration of vancomycin and fluoroquinolones (grade 1A). Select appropriate agents based on the surgical procedure, most common pathogens causing SSI, for specific procedure and follow published recommendation. [194, 195] Discontinue prophylaxis within 24 hours after most surgical procedures. For cardiac procedures continue for 48 hours.
2 It is recommended that only hair that will interfere with the operation be removed, and that if hair removal is necessary, then it should be removed by using electric clippers (grade 1B).
3 Blood glucose levels during the immediate postoperative period for patients undergoing cardiac surgery: should be<200 mg/dL on postoperative day 1 and postoperative day 2, with procedure day being postoperative day 0 (grade 1C).
4 Identify and treat infections remote to the surgical site before elective surgery (grade 1B).
5 Measurement of rates of compliance as well as feedback to providers about the above recommendation adherence is important. (A-III)
6 Delineate Institutional/hospital policies and practices targeting reduction in the risk of SSI in line with evidence-based standards (e.g., Centers for Disease Control and Prevention and professional organization guidelines) (A-II). [175]
7 Education of surgical providers and perioperative personnel about SSI prevention regarding risk factors, local data including epidemiology and prevalence of resistant organisms and Education of patients and their families are all among important preventive measures.

Clostridium Difficile Infection (CDI)

Despite increasing awareness and interventions for prevention of Clostridium *difficile* Infections, rates of CDI continue to rise. It is now along with Methicillin resistant Staphylococcus aureus (MRSA) the most common organism to cause healthcare-associated infections in the United States. [196]

There are numerous reports of an increase in CDI severity mainly associated with the BI/NAP1/027 strain of C. difficile. [196]. This strain produces more of both toxins A and B in vitro than other strains of C. *difficile*, produces a third kind of toxin called the binary toxin, and is highly resistant to fluoroquinolones. CDI results in increased length of hospital stay, costs, morbidity, and mortality among adult patients.US hospitals spends close to $3.5 billion per year on CDI. CDI has been associated with an attributable mortality rate of 6.9% at 30 days post diagnosis and 16.7% at 1 year after diagnosis. [196]

Clostridium difficile infection (CDI) is the most common infectious cause of diarrhea in the ICU [197]. The changing CDI epidemiology has had a significant impact in the ICU setting. The incidence as well as the severity of CDI is increasing in the ICU [198].There are increased number of admissions to the ICU for the management of complications from CDI [199]. The most common risk factors identified for CDI include antibiotic exposure, age > 60 years, longer duration of hospital stay, severe underlying disease, and gastric acid suppression. e.g that caused by PPI use [200].

Many of these factors are present in critically ill patients residing in the ICU, making it unsurprising that ICU stay is in itself a risk factor [201]. Almost all antibiotics have been associated with CDI. Cephalosporins, ampicillin, and clindamycin remain important predisposing antibiotics 95% of patients with CDI have had prior antibiotic therapy. PPI use, enteral feeding and mechanical ventilation are other contributing factors for development of CDI.

Survival of C. Difficile in the Healthcare Environment

C. difficile is a fastidious anaerobe and the vegetative cell usually dies within 24 hours, outside the colon. [202, 203] However, *C. difficile* produces spores that can live in the environment for many months and are highly resistant to cleaning and disinfection measures. [204] The spores make it possible for the organism to survive passage through the stomach, resisting killing by gastric acid, when ingested. After ingestion, the spores can germinate, produce toxins, and cause disease.Both the vegetative and spore forms of *C. difficile* need to be targeted with environmental cleaning and disinfection.

Transmission of C. Difficile to Patients from the Healthcare Environment

The two major reservoirs of *C. difficile* in healthcare settings are infected humans (symptomatic or asymptomatic) and inanimate objects. Patients with symptomatic intestinal infection are thought to be the major reservoir. [205]

The level of environmental contamination with *C. difficile* spores increases with increasing severity of disease in the patient. [206] However, asymptomatic colonized patients should also be considered as a potential source of contamination and transmission [206] Patient care items such as electronic thermometers and contaminated commodes have been implicated in the transmission of CDI. [207] Transmission of *C. difficile* to the patient on health care providers' hands is thought to be the most likely mode of transmission strongly suggested by the fact that these of gloves can reduce rates of CDI. Alcohol is not effective in killing *C. difficile* spores, but use of alcohol-based hand rubs (ABHR) has not shown an increase in CDI rates over hand washing. With increased rates or in an outbreak situation, it is better to wash hands with soap and water when caring for patients with known CDI.8 Transmission of many diseases including CDI has been known to occur from contaminated mobile telephones. [9]

Transmission Via Patient Care Activities

There are a number of patient care activities that provide an opportunity for transmission of *C. difficile*. Some of these activities include:

- Sharing of electronic thermometers that have been used for obtaining rectal temperatures (handles may be contaminated with *C. difficile* even through probes are changed and probe covers used)
- Oral care or oral suctioning when hands or items are contaminated
- Administration of feedings or medication
- Emergency procedures such as intubation
- Poor hand hygiene practices
- Sharing of patient care items without appropriate disinfection
- Ineffective environmental cleaning

Consideration of methods of transmission and interrupting these are important strategies along with preventive strategies. Strict adherence to hand hygiene. is essential for the prevention of CDI. Common antimicrobial agents (including alcohols, chlorhexidine, hexachlorophene, iodophors, PCMX, and triclosan) are not active against spores; but, soap and water hand washing mechanically removes *C. difficile* spores from hands of providers when compared to ABHRs. [1,2] There have been no studies in acute care settings that demonstrate an increase in CDI with ABHRs or a decrease in rates of CDI with traditional hand washing with soap and water. The use of soap and water for hand hygiene is not preferred over the use of ABHRs after caring for a patient with CDI in non-outbreak setting. The recommendation to use soap and water preferentially in outbreak settings after caring for a patient with CDI is recommended based on the theoretical benefit of the physical removal and dilution of spores from the hands by washing, rather than killing the spores. [202]

According to the CDC Healthcare Infection Control Practices Advisory Committee (HICPAC) hand hygiene guideline, the hands of health care providers are frequently contaminated with *C. difficile* following patient contact. Wearing gloves can significantly reduce the spread of *C. difficile* by providing a physical barrier that decreases, if not prevents, hand contamination with spores.4 Gloves should be removed if the integrity is compromised. The gloves should be removed properly to prevent hand contamination. After gloves are removed, the Health Care Providers' hands should be washed with a nonantimicrobial or an antimicrobial soap and water or disinfected with an ABHR [204]. Although some facilities remove ABHR from a patient's room if the patient has CDI, removing ABHRs may increase the risk of other infections. The use of ABHRs has been shown to improve compliance and reduce the risk of multidrug-resistant organisms (MDROs) such as vancomycin-resistant *Enterococcus* and MRSA. When providing device-related care where there is a need to decontaminate hands and wear clean gloves, ABHRs may improve compliance, minimize the time for cleaning hands, and reduce the risk of device-related infections.

In an intensive care unit (ICU) study it was noted that hand hygiene compliance was the lowest after brief encounters lasting less than 2 minutes. The brief encounters made up a substantial portion of the contact where the providers had opportunities for washing hands. The results of this study show that it is important to improve adherence with hand hygiene even for brief encounters since there is significant contamination and impact on transmission even with brief encounter.

Association for Professionals in Infection Control and Epidemiology recommend advanced technologies to monitor hand hygiene electronically any time a provider enters the room. Electronic devices can be used to provide information on frequency, time, and location of its use, and also reveal trends in hand disinfection events over time. These can be employed in addition to direct observations.

Antibiotic Resistance and Emerging Infections Program

Each year in the United States, at least 2 million people become infected with bacteria that are resistant to antibiotics and at least 23,000 people die each year as a direct result of these infections. Many more people die from other conditions that are complicated by antibiotic-resistant infections. [212] Antibiotic-resistant infections can occur anywhere. Data show that most occur in the general community; however, most deaths related to antibiotic resistance occur in the healthcare settings such as hospitals and nursing homes. [212] A threat assessment classifies resistant organisms into the following categories.

Hazard Level -- Urgent

These are high-consequence antibiotic-resistant threats because of significant risks identified across several criteria. These threats may not be currently widespread but have the potential to become so and require urgent public health attention to identify o limit transmission. They include *Clostridium difficile* (*C. difficile*), Carbapenem-resistant Enterobacteriaceae (CRE), Drug-resistant *Neisseria gonorrhea* (cephalosporin resistance)

Hazard Level -- Serious

These are significant antibiotic-resistance threats.For varying reasons (e.g., low or declining domestic incidence or reasonable availability of therapeutic agents), they are not considered urgent, but these threats will worsen and may become urgent without ongoing public health monitoring and prevention activities.

Multidrug-resistant *Acinetobacter*, Drug-resistant Campylobacter, Fluconazole-resistant *Candida species*, Extended spectrum β-lactamase producing Enterobacteriaceae (ESBLs), Vancomycin-resistant *Enterococcus* (VRE), Multidrug-resistant *Pseudomonas aeruginosa*, Drug-resistant Non-typhoidal *Salmonella*, Drug-resistant *Salmonella* Typhi, Drug-resistant *Shigella*, Methicillin-resistant *Staphylococcus aureus* (MRSA), Drug-resistant *Streptococcus pneumoniae*, Drug-resistant tuberculosis (MDR and XDR) are included in this category.

Hazard Level -- Concerning

These are bacteria for which the threat of antibiotic resistance is low, and/ or there are multiple therapeutic options for resistant infections. These bacterial pathogens cause severe illness. Threats in this category require monitoring and in some cases rapid incident or outbreak response.

Vancomycin-resistant *Staphylococcus aureus* (VRSA), Erythromycin-resistant *Streptococcus* Group A, Clindamycin-resistant Streptococcus Group B are among the pathogens in this category.

CDC recommends 4 core strategies to manage Antibiotic drug resistance.

1 Developing new Drugs and Diagnostic Tests. Because antibiotic resistance occurs as part of a natural process in which bacteria evolve, it can be slowed but not stopped. Therefore, we will always need new antibiotics to keep up with resistant bacteria as well as new diagnostic tests to track the development of resistance.
2 Preventing Infections, Preventing the Spread of Resistance. Avoiding infections in the first place reduces the amount of antibiotics that have to be used and reduces the likelihood that resistance will develop during therapy. There are many ways that drug-resistant infections can be prevented: immunization, safe food preparation, hand washing, and using antibiotics appropriately and only when necessary. In addition, preventing infections also prevents the spread of resistant bacteria.
3 Tracking. CDC gathers data on antibiotic-resistant infections, causes of infections and whether there are particular risk factors that cause some people to get resistant infections. With that information, experts can develop specific strategies to prevent those infections and prevent the resistant bacteria from spreading.
4 Improving Antibiotic Prescribing/Stewardship. Perhaps the single most important action needed to significantly slow down the development and spread of antibiotic-resistant infections is to change the way antibiotics are used. Up to half of antibiotic use in humans and much of antibiotic use in animals is unnecessary and inappropriate and makes everyone less safe. Stopping even some of the inappropriate and unnecessary use of antibiotics in people and animals would help greatly in slowing down the creation and spread of resistant bacteria. This commitment to always use antibiotics appropriately and safely, only when they are needed to treat disease, to choose the right antibiotics, to administer them in the right way in every case, is the corner stone of antibiotic stewardship.

Staff Education

1 Education of all Staff involved in patients with sepsis is highly recommended. Interactive, multifaceted, longitudinal educational programs, outreach and guideline implementation improve quality of care. [7] It has been seen that traditional methods of which are considered passive e.g., conferences, web sites, or didactic lectures, do not work as well as the interactive methodology (grade 1A).
2 Ongoing Educational initiatives to reduce healthcare-associated infection rates (grade 1C).
3 Surviving sepsis guidelines also recommend promotion of a culture of patient safety and individual accountability (grade 2D).

Every healthcare worker is responsible and accountable for ensuring patient safety; an essential component of it is infection prevention and control. [9, 10]

Appendix

Table 2. Strength of Recommendation and Quality of Evidence

Category/grade	Definition
Strength of recommendation	
A	Good evidence to support a recommendation for use
B	Moderate evidence to support a recommendation for use
C	Poor evidence to support a recommendation
Quality of evidence	
I	Evidence from ⩾1 properly randomized, controlled trial
II	Evidence from ⩾1 well-designed clinical trial, without randomization; from cohort or case-control analytic studies (preferably from >1 center); from multiple time series; or from dramatic results from uncontrolled experiments
III	Evidence from opinions of respected authorities, based on clinical experience, descriptive studies, or reports of expert committees

References

[1] Fridkin, S. K., Welbel, S. F., Weinstein, R. A. Magnitude and prevention of nosocomial infections in the intensive care unit. *Infect. Dis. Clin. North Am.* 1997; 11:479.

[2] Vincent, J. L., Rello, J., Marshall, J., et al. International study of the prevalence and outcomes of infection in intensive care units. *JAMA* 2009; 302:2323.

[3] Margaret Jean Hall, Ph.D.; Sonja N. Williams, M.P.H.; Carol J. De Frances, Ph.D.; and Aleksandr Golosinskiy, M. S. Inpatient Care for Septicemia or Sepsis: A Challenge for Patients and Hospitals, *NCHS Data Brief, No. 62*, June 2011.

[4] Chang, H. J., Lynm, C., Glass, R. M. Sepsis. *JAMA* 304(16):1856. 2010.

[5] Iwashyna, T. J., Ely, E. W., Smith, D. M., Langa, K. M. Long-term cognitive impairment and functional disability among survivors of severe sepsis. *JAMA* 304(16):1787–94. 2010.

[6] Dellinger, R. P., Levy, M. M., Rhodes, A., Annane, D., Gerlach, H., Opal, S. M., Sevransky, J. E., Sprung, C. L., Douglas, I. S., Jaeschke, R., Osborn, T. M., Nunnally, M. E., Townsend, S. R., Reinhart, K., Kleinpell, R. M., Angus, D. C., Deutschman, C. S., Machado, F. R., Rubenfeld, G. D., Webb, S. A., Beale, R. J., Vincent, J. L., Moreno, R.; Surviving Sepsis Campaign Guidelines Committee including the Pediatric Subgroup. Surviving sepsis campaign: international guidelines for management of severe sepsis and septic shock: 2012. *Crit. Care Med.* 2013 Feb.;41(2):580-637.

[7] Weinstein, R. A. Epidemiology and control of nosocomial infections in adult intensive care units. *Am. J. Med.* 1991; 91:179S.

[8] Kaye, K. S., Fraimow, H. S., Abrutyn, E. Pathogens resistant to antimicrobial agents. Epidemiology, molecular mechanisms, and clinical management. *Infect. Dis. Clin. North Am.* 2000; 14:293.

[9] Kaye, K. S., Marchaim, D., Smialowicz, C., Bentley, L. Suction regulators: a potential vector for hospital-acquired pathogens. *Infect. Control Hosp. Epidemiol.* 2010; 31:772.
[10] Baquero, F., Negri, M. C., Morosini, M. I., Blázquez, J. Antibiotic-selective environments. *Clin. Infect. Dis.* 1998; 27 Suppl. 1:S5.
[11] Bonten, M. J. Colonization pressure: a critical parameter in the epidemiology of antibiotic-resistant bacteria. *Crit. Care* 2012; 16:142.
[12] Ben-Ami, R., Rodríguez-Baño, J., Arslan, H., et al. A multinational survey of risk factors for infection with extended-spectrum beta-lactamase-producing enterobacteriaceae in nonhospitalized patients. *Clin. Infect. Dis.* 2009; 49:682.
[13] Safdar, N., Maki, D. G. The commonality of risk factors for nosocomial colonization and infection with antimicrobial-resistant Staphylococcus aureus, enterococcus, gram-negative bacilli, Clostridium difficile, and Candida. *Ann. Intern. Med.* 2002; 136:834.
[14] Kaye, K. S., Cosgrove, S., Harris, A., et al. Risk factors for emergence of resistance to broad-spectrum cephalosporins among Enterobacter spp. *Antimicrob. Agents Chemother.* 2001; 45:2628.
[15] National Nosocomial Infections Surveillance (NNIS) system report, data summary from January 1992-April 2000, issued June 2000. *Am. J. Infect. Control* 2000; 28:429.
[16] Hidron, A. I., Edwards, J. R., Patel, J., et al. NHSN annual update: antimicrobial-resistant pathogens associated with healthcare-associated infections: annual summary of data reported to the National Healthcare Safety Network at the Centers for Disease Control and Prevention, 2006-2007. *Infect. Control Hosp. Epidemiol.* 2008; 29:996.
[17] http://www.cdc.gov/hai/state-based/tracking.html.
[18] http://www.cdc.gov/nhsn/about.html.
[19] Mermel, L. A. Prevention of intravascular catheter-related infections. *Ann. Intern. Med.* 2000 Mar. 7;132(5):391-402. Erratum in: *Ann. Intern. Med.* 2000 Sep. 5;133(5):395.
[20] Centers for Disease Control and Prevention (CDC). Vital signs: central line-associated blood stream infections--United States, 2001, 2008, and 2009. *MMWR Morb. Mortal Wkly Rep.* 2011; 60:243.
[21] Wisplinghoff, H., Bischoff, T., Tallent, S. M., et al. Nosocomial bloodstream infections in US hospitals: analysis of 24,179 cases from a prospective nationwide surveillance study. *Clin. Infect. Dis.* 2004; 39: 309.
[22] Pittet, D., Li, N., Woolson, R. F., Wenzel, R. P. Microbiological factors influencing the outcome of nosocomial bloodstream infections: a 6-year validated, population-based model. *Clin. Infect. Dis.* 1997; 24:1068.
[23] Warren, D. K., Quadir, W. W., Hollenbeak, C. S., et al. Attributable cost of catheter-associated bloodstream infection among intensive care patients in a nonteaching hospital. *Crit. Care Med.* 2006; 34:2084-2089.
[24] Kluger, D. M., Maki, D. G. The relative risk of intravascular device related bloodstream infections in adults [Abstract]. In: *Abstracts of the 39th Interscience Conference on Antimicrobial Agents and Chemo-therapy.* San Francisco, CA: American Society for Microbiology, 1999: 514.
[25] Digiovine, B., Chenoweth, C., Watts, C., Higgins, M. The attributable mortality and costs of primary nosocomial bloodstream infections in the intensive care unit. *Am. J. Respir. Crit. Care Med.* 1999;160:976--81.

[26] Rello, J., Ochagavia, A., Sabanes, E., et al. Evaluation of outcome of intravenous catheter-related infections in critically ill patients. *Am. J. Respir. Crit. Care Med.* 2000;162:1027--30.

[27] Soufir, L., Timsit, J. F., Mahe, C., Carlet, J., Regnier, B., Chevret, S. Attributable morbidity and mortality of catheter-related septicemia in critically ill patients: a matched, risk-adjusted, cohort study. *Infect. Control Hosp. Epidemiol.* 1999;20:396--401.

[28] Collignon, P. J. Intravascular catheter associated sepsis: a common problem. The Australian Study on Intravascular Catheter Associated Sepsis. *Med. J. Aust.* 1994;161:374--8.

[29] Pittet, D., Tarara, D., Wenzel, R. P. Nosocomial bloodstream infection in critically ill patients. Excess length of stay, extra costs, and attributable mortality. *JAMA* 1994;271:1598--601.

[30] A compendium of strategies to prevent healthcare-associated infections in acute care hospitals. Yokoe, D. S., Mermel, L. A., Anderson, D. J., Arias, K. M., Burstin, H., Calfee, D. P., Coffin, S. E., Dubberke, E. R., Fraser, V., Gerding, D. N., Griffin, F. A., Gross, P., Kaye, K. S., Klompas, M., Lo, E., Marschall, J., Nicolle, L., Pegues, D. A., Perl, T. M., Podgorny, K., Saint, S., Salgado, C. D., Weinstein, R. A., Wise, R., Classen. *Infect. Control Hosp. Epidemiol.* 2008 Oct.; 29 Suppl. 1:S12-21.

[31] Dimick, J. B., Pelz, R. K., Consunji, R., Swoboda, S. M., Hendrix, C. W., Lipsett, P. A. Increased resource use associated with catheter-related bloodstream infection in the surgical intensive care unit. *Arch. Surg.* 2001;136:229--34.

[32] CDC. National Nosocomial Infections Surveillance (NNIS) System report, data summary from January 1990--May 1999, issued June 1999. *Am. J. Infect. Control* 1999;27:520--32.

[33] Joint Commission on the Accreditation of Healthcare Organizations. Accreditation manual for hospitals. In: *Joint Commission on the Accreditation of Healthcare Organizations,* ed. Chicago, IL: Joint Commission on the Accreditation of Healthcare Organizations, 1994: 121--40.

[34] CDC. National Nosocomial Infections Surveillance (NNIS) System report, data summary from January 1992--June 2001, issued August 2001. *Am. J. Infect. Control* 2001;6:404--21.

[35] Fridkin, S. K., Pear, S. M., Williamson, T. H., Galgiani, J. N., Jarvis, W. R. The role of understaffing in central venous catheter-associated bloodstream infections. *Infect. Control Hosp. Epidemiol.* 1996;17:150--8.

[36] Alonso-Echanove, J., Edwards, J. R., Richards, M. J., et al. Effect of nurse staffing and antimicrobial-impregnated central venous catheters on the risk for bloodstream infections in intensive care units. Infect. Control Hosp. Epidemiol. 2003;24:916-25.

[37] Robert, J., Fridkin, S. K., Blumberg, H. M., et al. The influence of the composition of the nursing staff on primary bloodstream infection rates in a surgical intensive care unit. Infect. Control Hosp. Epidemiol. 2000; 21:12-7.

[38] Mian, N. Z., Bayly, R., Schreck, D. M., Besserman, E. B., Richmand, D. Incidence of deep venous thrombosis associated with femoral venous catheterization. Acad. Emerg. Med. 1997;4:1118-21.

[39] Merrer, J., De Jonghe, B., Golliot, F., et al. Complications of femoral and subclavian venous catheterization in critically ill patients: a randomized controlled trial. JAMA 2001;286:700-7.

[40] Goetz, A. M., Wagener, M. M., Miller, J. M., Muder, R. R. Risk of infection due to central venous catheters: effect of site of placement and catheter type. Infect. Control Hosp. Epidemiol. 1998;19:842-5.

[41] Maki, D. G., Mermel, L. A. Infections due to infusion therapy. In: Bennett, J. V., Brachman, P. S., eds. *Hospital Infections.* 4th ed. Philadelphia: Lippencott-Raven, 1998:689--724.

[42] Richet, H., Hubert, B., Nitemberg, G., et al. Prospective multicenter study of vascular-catheter-related complications and risk factors for positive central-catheter cultures in intensive care unit patients. *J. Clin. Microbiol.* 1990;28:2520--5.

[43] Maki, D. G., Goldman, D. A., Rhame, F. S. Infection control in intravenous therapy. Ann. Intern. Med. 1973;79:867-87.

[44] Band, J. D., Maki, D. G. Steel needles used for intravenous therapy. Morbidity in patients with hematologic malignancy. Arch. Intern. Med. 1980;140:31.

[45] Hilton, E., Haslett, T. M., Borenstein, M. T., Tucci, V., Isenberg, H. D., Singer, C. Central catheter infections: single- versus triple-lumen catheters. Influence of guide wires on infection rates when used for replacement of catheters. Am. J. Med. 1988;84:667-72.

[46] Yeung, C., May, J., Hughes, R. Infection rate for single lumen v triple lumen subclavian catheters. Infect. Control Hosp. Epidemiol. 1988;9: 154-8.

[47] Maki, D. G., Ringer, M., Alvarado, C. J. Prospective randomised trial of povidone-iodine, alcohol, and chlorhexidine for prevention of infection associated with central venous and arterial catheters. Lancet 1991;338: 339-43.

[48] Mimoz, O., Pieroni, L., Lawrence, C., et al. Prospective, randomized trial of two antiseptic solutions for prevention of central venous or arterial catheter colonization and infection in intensive care unit patients. Crit. Care Med. 1996;24:1818-23.

[49] Zakrzewska-Bode, A., Muytjens, H. L., Liem, K. D., Hoogkamp-Korstanje, J. A. Mupirocin resistance in coagulase-negative staphylococci, after topical prophylaxis for the reduction of colonization of central venous catheters. J. Hosp. Infect. 1995;31:189-93.

[50] Zakrzewska-Bode, A., Muytjens, H. L., Liem, K. D., Hoogkamp-Korstanje, J. A. Mupirocin resistance in coagulase-negative staphylo-cocci, after topical prophylaxis for the reduction of colonization of central venous catheters. *J. Hosp. Infect.* 1995;31:189-93.

[51] Bleasdale, S. C., Trick, W. E., Gonzalez, I. M., Lyles, R. D., Hayden, M. K., Weinstein, R. A. Effectiveness of chlorhexidine bathing to reduce catheter-associated bloodstream infections in medical intensive care unit patients. Arch. Intern. Med. 2007;167:2073-9.

[52] Munoz-Price, L. S., Hota, B., Stemer, A., Weinstein, R. A. Prevention of bloodstream infections by use of daily chlorhexidine baths for patients at a long-term acute care hospital. Infect. Control Hosp. Epidemiol. 2009; 30:1031-5.

[53] Popovich, K. J., Hota, B., Hayes, R., Weinstein, R. A., Hayden, M. K. Effectiveness of routine patient cleansing with chlorhexidine gluconate for infection prevention in the medical intensive care unit. Infect. Control Hosp. Epidemiol. 2009;30:959-63.

[54] Yamamoto, A. J., Solomon, J. A., Soulen, M. C., et al. Sutureless securement device reduces complications of peripherally inserted central venous catheters. *J. Vasc. Interv. Radiol.* 2002;13:77-81.

[55] Brun-Buisson, C., Doyon, F., Sollet, J. P., Cochard, J. F., Cohen, Y., Nitenberg, G. Prevention of intravascular catheter-related infection with newer chlorhexidine-silver sulfadiazine-coated catheters: a randomized controlled trial. *Intensive Care Med.* 2004;30:837-43.

[56] Ostendorf, T., Meinhold, A., Harter, C., et al. Chlorhexidine and silver-sulfadiazine coated central venous catheters in haematological patients–a double-blind, randomised, prospective, controlled trial. *Support Care Cancer* 2005;13:993-1000.

[57] Rupp, M. E., Lisco, S. J., Lipsett, P. A., et al. Effect of a second-generation venous catheter impregnated with chlorhexidine and silver sulfadiazine on central catheter-related infections: a randomized, controlled trial. *Ann. Intern. Med.* 2005;143:570-80.

[58] Darouiche, R. O., Raad, I. I., Heard, S. O., et al. A comparison of two antimicrobial-impregnated central venous catheters. Catheter Study Group. *N. Engl. J. Med.* 1999;340:1-8.

[59] Raad, I., Darouiche, R., Dupuis, J., et al. Central venous catheters coated with minocycline and rifampin for the prevention of catheter-related colonization and bloodstream infections. A randomized, double-blind trial. The Texas Medical Center Catheter Study Group. *Ann. Intern. Med.* 1997;127:267-74.

[60] Hanna, H., Benjamin, R., Chatzinikolaou, I., et al. Long-term silicone central venous catheters impregnated with minocycline and rifampin decrease rates of catheter-related bloodstream infection in cancer patients: a prospective randomized clinical trial. J. Clin. Oncol. 2004;22: 3163-71.

[61] Bhutta, A., Gilliam, C., Honeycutt, M., et al. Reduction of bloodstream infections associated with catheters in paediatric intensive care unit: stepwise approach. BMJ 2007;334:362.

[62] Chelliah, A., Heydon, K. H., Zaoutis, T. E., et al. Observational trial of antibiotic-coated central venous catheters in critically ill pediatric patients. Pediatr. Infect. Dis. J. 2007;26:816-20.

[63] Van de Wetering, M. D., van Woensel, J. B. M. Prophylactic antibioticsfor preventing early central venous catheter Gram positive infectionsin oncology patients. *Cochrane Database of Systematic Reviews* 2007; Issue 1.

[64] O'Grady, N. P., Alexander, M., Burns, L. A., Dellinger, E. P., Garland, J., Heard, S. O., Lipsett, P. A., Masur, H., Mermel, L. A., Pearson, M. L., Raad, I. I., Randolph, A. G., Rupp, M. E., Saint, S.; Healthcare Infection Control Practices Advisory Committee (HICPAC). Guidelines for the prevention of intravascular catheter-related infections. *Clin. Infect. Dis.* 2011 May;52(9):e162-93.

[65] Henrickson, K. J., Axtell, R. A., Hoover, S. M., et al. Prevention of central venous catheter-related infections and thrombotic events in immunocompromised children by the use of vancomycin/ ciprofloxacin/ heparin flush solution: a randomized, multicenter, double-blind trial. *J. Clin. Oncol.* 2000; 18:1269–78.

[66] Garland, J. S., Alex, C. P., Henrickson, K. J., McAuliffe, T. L., Maki, D. G. A vancomycin-heparin lock solution for prevention of nosocomial bloodstream infection in critically ill neonates with peripherally inserted central venous catheters: a prospective, randomized trial. *Pediatrics* 2005; 116:e198–205.

[67] Daghistani, D., Horn, M., Rodriguez, Z., Schoenike, S., Toledano, S. Prevention of indwelling central venous catheter sepsis. *Med. Pediatr. Oncol.* 1996; 26:405–8.

[68] Barriga, F. J., Varas, M., Potin, M., et al. Efficacy of a vancomycin solution to prevent bacteremia associated with an indwelling central venous catheter in neutropenic and non-neutropenic cancer patients. *Med. Pediatr. Oncol.* 1997; 28:196–200.

[69] Dogra, G. K., Herson, H., Hutchison, B., et al. Prevention of tunneled hemodialysis catheter-related infections using catheter-restricted filling with gentamicin and citrate: a randomized controlled study. *J. Am. Soc. Nephrol.* 2002; 13:2133–9.

[70] Allon, M. Prophylaxis against dialysis catheter-related bacteremia with a novel antimicrobial lock solution. *Clin. Infect. Dis.* 2003; 36:1539–44.

[71] Elhassan, N. O., Stevens, T. P., Gigliotti, F., Hardy, D. J., Cole, C. A., Sinkin, R. A. Vancomycin usage in central venous catheters in a neonatal intensive care unit. *Pediatr. Infect. Dis. J.* 2004; 23:201–6.

[72] McIntyre, C. W., Hulme, L. J., Taal, M., Fluck, R. J. Locking of tunneled hemodialysis catheters with gentamicin and heparin. *Kidney Int.* 2004; 66:801–5.

[73] Betjes, M. G., van Agteren, M. Prevention of dialysis catheter-related sepsis with a citrate-taurolidine-containing lock solution. *Nephrol. Dial. Transplant.* 2004; 19:1546–1.

[74] Weijmer, M. C., van den Dorpel, M. A., Van de Ven, P. J., et al. Randomized,clinical trial comparison of trisodium citrate 30% and heparin as catheter-locking solution in hemodialysis patients. *J. Am. Soc. Nephrol.*, 2005; 16:2769–77.

[75] Bleyer, A. J., Mason, L., Russell, G., Raad, I. I., Sherertz, R. J. A randomized, controlled trial of a new vascular catheter flush solution (minocycline-EDTA) in temporary hemodialysis access. *Infect. Control Hosp. Epidemiol.* 2005; 26:520–4.

[76] Kim, S. H., Song, K. I., Chang, J. W., et al. Prevention of uncuffed hemodialysis, catheter-related bacteremia using an antibiotic lock technique:a prospective, randomized clinical trial. *Kidney Int.* 2006; 69: 161–4.

[77] Al-Hwiesh, A. K., Abdul-Rahman, I. S. Successful prevention of tunneled, central catheter infection by antibiotic lock therapy using vancomycin and gentamycin. *Saudi J. Kidney Dis. Transpl.* 2007; 18: 239–47.

[78] Jurewitsch, B., Lee, T., Park, J., Jeejeebhoy, K. Taurolidine 2% as an antimicrobial lock solution for prevention of recurrent catheter-related bloodstream infections. *J. Parenter. Enteral Nutr.* 1998; 22:242–4.

[79] Darouiche, R. O., Raad, I. I., Heard, S. O., et al.: A comparison of two antimicrobial-impregnated central venous catheters. Catheter Study Group. *N. Engl. J. Med.* 1999; 340:1–8.

[80] Boo, N. Y., Wong, N. C., Zulkifli, S. S., Lye, M. S. Risk factors associated withumbilical vascular catheter-associated thrombosis in newborn infants. *J. Paediatr. Child Health* 1999; 35:460–5.

[81] Avila-Figueroa, C., Goldmann, D. A., Richardson, D. K., et al.: Intravenous lipid emulsions are the major determinant of coagulase-negative staphylococcal bacteremia in very low birth weight newborns. *Pediatr. Infect. Dis. J.* 1998; 17:10–17.

[82] Crocker, K. S., Noga, R., Filibeck, D. J., et al.: Microbial growth comparisons of five commercial parenteral lipid emulsions. *JPEN J. Parenter. Enteral Nutr.* 1984; 8:391–395.

[83] Hanna, H. A., Raad, I.: Blood products: A significant risk factor for long-term catheter-related bloodstream infections in cancer patients. *Infect. Control Hosp. Epidemiol.* 2001; 22:165–166.

[84] Jarvis, W. R., Highsmith, A. K.: Bacterial growth and endotoxin production in lipid emulsion. *J. Clin. Microbiol.* 1984; 19:17–20.

[85] Raad, I., Hanna, H. A., Awad, A., et al.: Optimal frequency of changing intravenous administration sets: is it safe to prolong use beyond 72 hours? *Infect. Control Hosp. Epidemiol.* 2001; 22:136–139.

[86] Saiman, L., Ludington, E., Dawson, J. D., et al.: Risk factors for Candida species colonization of neonatal intensive care unit patients. *Pediatr. Infect. Dis. J.* 2001; 20:1119–1124.

[87] American Thoracic Society, Infectious Diseases Society of America. Guidelines for the management of adults with hospital-acquired, ventilator-associated, and healthcare-associated pneumonia. *Am. J. Respir. Crit. Care Med.* 2005; 171:388.

[88] Coffin, S. E., Klompas, M., Classen, D., et al. Strategies to prevent ventilator-associated pneumonia in acute care hospitals. *Infect. Control Hosp. Epidemiol.* 2008; 29 Suppl. 1:S31.

[89] Safdar, N., Dezfulian, C., Collard, H. R., et al.: Clinical and economic consequences of ventilator-associated pneumonia: A systematic review. *Crit. Care Med.* 2005; 33:2184–2193.

[90] Cook, D. J., Walter, S. D., Cook, R. J., et al.: Incidence of and risk factors for ventilator-associated pneumonia in critically ill patients. *Ann. Intern. Med.* 1998; 129:433–440.

[91] Tejerina, E., Frutos-Vivar, F., Restrepo, M. I., et al.: Incidence, risk factors, and outcome of ventilator-associated pneumonia. *J. Crit. Care* 2006; 21:56–65.

[92] Warren, D. K., Shukla, S. J., Olsen, M. A., et al.: Outcome and attributable cost of ventilator-associated pneumonia among intensive care unit patients in a suburban medical center. *Crit. Care Med.* 2003; 31:1312–1317.

[93] Lai, K., Baker, S., Fontecchio, S.: Impact of a program of intensive surveillance and interventions targeting ventilated patients in the reduction of ventilator-associated pneumonia and its cost-effectiveness. *Infect. Control Hosp. Epidemiol.* 2003; 24:859–863.

[94] Zack, J. E., Garrison, T., Trovillion, E., et al.: Effect of an education program aimed at reducing the occurrence of ventilator-associated pneumonia. *Crit. Care Med.* 2002; 30:2407–2412.

[95] Lorente, L., Blot, S., Rello, J.: Evidence on measures for the prevention of ventilator-associated pneumonia. *Eur. Respir. J.* 2007; 30:1193–1207.

[96] Wip, C., Napolitano, L.: Bundles to prevent ventilator-associated pneumonia: how valuable are they? *Curr. Opin. Infect. Dis.* 2009; 22: 159–166.

[97] Muscedere, J., Dodek, P., Keenan, S., et al.: Comprehensive evidence-based clinical practice guidelines for ventilator-associated pneumonia: Diagnosis and treatment. *J. Crit. Care* 2008; 23:138–147.
[98] Huxley, E. J., Viroslav, J., Gray, W. R., et al.: Pharyngeal aspiration in normal adults and patients with depressed consciousness. *Am. J. Med.* 1978; 64:564–568.
[99] Drakulovic, M. B., Torres, A., Bauer, T. T., et al.: Supine body position as a risk factor for nosocomial pneumonia in mechanically ventilated patients: A randomised trial. *Lancet* 1999; 354:1851–1858.
[100] Fernández-Crehuet, R., Díaz-Molina, C., de Irala, J., et al.: Nosocomial infection in an intensive-care unit: Identification of risk factors. *Infect. Control Hosp. Epidemiol.* 1997; 18:825–830.
[101] Kollef, M. H.: Ventilator-associated pneumonia. A multivariate analysis. *JAMA* 1993; 270:1965–1970.
[102] Song, H. J., Liu, J. T., Gao, S. Q., et al.: Clinical investigation on the compliance and the validity of ventilator bundle. *Zhongguo Wei Zhong Bing Ji Jiu Yi Xue* 2009; 21:660–663.
[103] Van Nieuwenhoven, C. A., Vandenbroucke-Grauls, C., van Tiel, F. H., et al.: Feasibility and effects of the semirecumbent position to prevent ventilator-associated pneumonia: A randomized study. *Crit. Care Med.* 2006; 34:396–402.
[104] Cason, C. L., Tyner, T., Saunders, S., et al.: Nurses' implementation of guidelines for ventilator-associated pneumonia from the Centers for Disease Control and Prevention. *Am. J. Crit. Care* 2007; 16:28–36.
[105] Dezfulian, C., Shojania, K., Collard, H. R., et al.: Subglottic secretion drainage for preventing ventilator-associated pneumonia: A meta-analysis. *Am. J. Med.* 2005; 118:11–18.
[106] Kollef, M. H., Afessa, B., Anzueto, A., et al.: Silver-coated endotracheal tubes and incidence of ventilator-associated pneumonia: The NASCENT randomized trial. *JAMA* 2008; 300:805–813.
[107] Rello, J., Kollef, M., Diaz, E., et al.: Reduced burden of bacterial airway colonization with a novel silver-coated endotracheal tube in a randomized multiple-center feasibility study. *Crit. Care Med.* 2006; 34: 2766–2772.
[108] Poelaert, J., Depuydt, P., De Wolf, A., et al.: Polyurethane cuffed endotracheal tubes to prevent early postoperative pneumonia after cardiac surgery: A pilot study. *J. Thoracic. Cardiovasc. Surg.* 2008; 135: 771–776.
[109] Rello, J., Soñora, R., Jubert, P., et al.: Pneumonia in intubated patients: Role of respiratory airway care. *Am. J. Respir. Crit. Care Med.* 1996; 154:111–115.
[110] Niël-Weise, B. S., Wille, J. C., van den Broek, P. J.: Humidification policies for mechanically ventilated intensive care patients and prevention of ventilator-associated pneumonia: A systematic review of randomized controlled trials. *J. Hosp. Infect.* 2007; 65:285–291.
[111] Davis, K. Jr, Evans, S. L., Campbell, R. S., et al.: Prolonged use of heat and moisture exchangers does not affect device efficiency or frequency rate of nosocomial pneumonia. *Crit. Care Med.* 2000; 28:1412–1418.
[112] Thomachot, L., Leone, M., Razzouk, K., et al.: Randomized clinical trial of extended use of a hydrophobic condenser humidifier: 1 vs. 7 days. *Crit. Care Med.* 2002; 30:232–237.

[113] Thomson, L., Morton, R., Cuthbertson, S., et al.: Tracheal suctioning of adults with an artificial airway. *Best Practice* 2000; 4:1–6.
[114] Celik, S. S., Elbas, N. O.: The standard of suction for patients undergoing endotracheal intubation. *Intensive Crit. Care Nurs.* 2000; 16: 191–198.
[115] Rolls, K., Smith, K., Jones, P., et al.: Suctioning an adult with a tracheal tube. *NSW Health Statewide Guidelines for Intensive Care*. New South Wales Health, Sydney, 2007.
[116] Wood, C. J.: Endotracheal suctioning: A literature review. *Intensive Crit. Care Nurs.* 1998; 14:124–136.
[117] Pedersen, C. M., Rosendahl-Nielsen, M., Hjermind, J., et al.: Endotracheal suctioning of the adult intubated patient—What is the evidence? *Intensive Crit. Care Nurs.* 2009; 25:21–30.
[118] Torres, A., el-Ebiary, M., González, J., et al.: Gastric and pharyngeal flora in nosocomial pneumonia acquired during mechanical ventilation. *Am. Rev. Respir. Dis.* 1993; 148:352–357.
[119] Vallés, J., Artigas, A., Rello, J., et al.: Continuous aspiration of subglottic secretions in preventing ventilator-associated pneumonia. *Ann. Intern. Med.* 1995; 122:179–186.
[120] Abele-Horn, M., Dauber, A., Bauernfeind, A., et al.: Decrease in nosocomial pneumonia in ventilated patients by selective oropharyngeal decontamination (SOD). *Intensive Care Med.* 1997; 23:187–195.
[121] Torres, A., el-Ebiary, M., González, J., et al.: Gastric and pharyngeal flora in nosocomial pneumonia acquired during mechanical ventilation. *Am. Rev. Respir. Dis.* 1993; 148:352–357.
[122] Vallés, J., Artigas, A., Rello, J., et al.: Continuous aspiration of subglottic secretions in preventing ventilator-associated pneumonia. *Ann. Intern. Med.* 1995; 122:179–186.
[123] Abele-Horn, M., Dauber, A., Bauernfeind, A., et al.: Decrease in nosocomial pneumonia in ventilated patients by selective oropharyngeal decontamination (SOD). *Intensive Care Med.* 1997; 23:187–195.
[124] Johanson, W. G. Jr, Seidenfeld, J. J., de los Santos, R., et al.: Prevention of nosocomial pneumonia using topical and parenteral antimicrobial agents. *Am. Rev. Respir. Dis.* 1988; 137:265–272.
[125] Berry, A., Davidson, P.: Consensus-based clinical guideline for the provision of oral care for the critically ill adult. *NSW Health Statewide Guidelines for Intensive Care.* New South Wales Health, Sydney, 2007.
[126] Fields, L. B.: Oral care intervention to reduce incidence of ventilator-associated pneumonia in the neurologic intensive care unit. *J. Neurosci. Nurs.* 2008; 40:291–298.
[127] Garcia, R., Jendresky, L., Colbert, L., et al.: Reducing ventilator-associated pneumonia through advanced oral-dental care: A 48-month study. *Am. J. Crit. Care* 2009; 18:523–532.
[128] Munro, C. L., Grap, M. J., Jones, D. J., et al.: Chlorhexidine, toothbrushing, and preventing ventilator-associated pneumonia in critically ill adults. *Am. J. Crit. Care* 2009; 18:428–437.
[129] Weireter, L., Collins, J., et al.: Impact of a monitored program of care on incidence of ventilator-associated pneumonia: results of a longterm performance-improvement project. *J. Am. Coll Surg.* 2009; 208:700–704; discussion 704–705.

[130] Ross, A., Crumpler, J.: The impact of an evidence-based practice education program on the role of oral care in the prevention of ventilator-associated pneumonia. *Intensive Crit. Care Nurs.* 2007; 23: 132–136.

[131] Blot, S., Vandijck, D., Labeau, S.: Oral care of intubated patients. *Clin. Pulmonary Med.* 2008; 15:153–160.

[132] Grap, M. J., Munro, C. L., Ashtiani, B., et al.: Oral care interventions in critical care: Frequency and documentation. *Am. J. Crit. Care* 2003; 12: 113–118.

[133] Jones, D. J., Munro, C. L.: Oral care and the risk of bloodstream infections in mechanically ventilated adults: A review. *Intensive Crit. Care Nurs.* 2008; 24:152–161.

[134] Munro, C. L., Grap, M. J.: Oral health and care in the intensive care unit: State of the science. *Am. J. Crit. Care* 2004; 13:25–33.

[135] Choo, A., Delac, D. M., Messer, L. B.: Oral hygiene measures and promotion: Review and considerations. *Aust. Dent. J.* 2001; 46:166–173.

[136] Moshrefi, A.: Chlorhexidine. *J. West Soc. Periodontol. Periodontal Abstr.* 2002; 50: 5–9.

[137] Fourrier, F., Cau-Pottier, E., Boutigny, H., et al.: Effects of dental plaque antiseptic decontamination on bacterial colonization and nosocomial infections in critically ill patients. *Intensive Care Med.* 2000; 26:1239–1247.

[138] DeRiso, A. J., Ladowski, J. S., Dillon, T. A., et al.: Chlorhexidine gluconate 0.12% oral rinse reduces the incidence of total nosocomial respiratory infection and nonprophylactic systemic antibiotic use in patients undergoing heart surgery. *Chest* 1996; 109:1556–1561.

[139] Chan, E. Y., Ruest, A., Meade, M. O., et al.: Oral decontamination for prevention of pneumonia in mechanically ventilated adults: Systematic review and meta-analysis. *BMJ* 2007; 334:889–893.

[140] Chlebicki, M. P., Safdar, N.: Topical chlorhexidine for prevention of ventilator-associated pneumonia: A meta-analysis. *Crit. Care Med.* 2007; 35:595–602.

[141] Tantipong, H., Morkchareonpong, C., Jaiyindee, S., et al.: Randomized controlled trial and meta-analysis of oral decontamination with 2% chlorhexidine solution for the prevention of ventilator-associated pneumonia. *Infect. Control Hosp. Epidemiol.* 2008; 29:131–136.

[142] Abidia, R. F.: Oral care in the intensive care unit: A review. *J. Contemp. Dent. Pract.* 2007; 8:76–82.

[143] Rello, J., Koulenti, D., Blot, S., et al.: Oral care practices in intensive care units: A survey of 59 European ICUs. *Intensive Care Med.* 2007; 33: 1066–1070.

[144] Galpern, D., Guerrero, A., Tu, A., et al.: Effectiveness of a central line bundle campaign on line-associated infections in the intensive care unit. *Surgery* 2008; 144:492–495.

[145] Alvarez-Lerma, F., ICU-acquired Pneumonia Study Group. Modification of empiric antibiotic treatment in patients with pneumonia acquiredin the intensive care unit. *Intensive Care Med.* 1996;22:387–394.

[146] Ibrahim, E. H., Ward, S., Sherman, G., Schaiff, R., Fraser, V. J., Kollef, M. H. Experience with a clinical guideline for the treatment of ventilatorassociate pneumonia. *Crit. Care Med.* 2001;29:1109–1115.

[147] Wood, G. C., Hanes, S. D., Croce, M. A., Fabian, T. C., Boucher, B. A. Comparison of ampicillin–sulbactam and imipenem–cilastatin for the treatment of*Acinetobacter* ventilator-associated pneumonia. *Clin. Infect. Dis.* 2002;34:1425–1430.

[148] Garnacho-Montero, J., Ortiz-Leyba, C., Jimenez-Jimenez, F. J., Barrero-Almodovar, A. E., Garcia-Garmendia, J. L., Bernabeu-WitteIl, M., Gallego-Lara, S. L., Madrazo-Osuna, J. Treatment of multidrug-resistant *Acinetobacter baumannii* ventilator-associated pneumonia (VAP) with intravenous colistin: a comparison with imipenem-susceptible. VAP. *Clin. Infect. Dis.* 2003;36:1111–1118.

[149] Paterson, D. L., Ko, W. C., Von Gottberg, A., Casellas, J. M., Mulazimoglu, L., Klugman, K. P., Bonomo, R. A., Rice, L. B., McCormack, J. G., Yu, V. L. Outcome of cephalosporin treatment for serious infections due to apparently susceptible organisms producing extended-spectrum _-lactamases: implications for the clinical microbiology laboratory. *J. Clin. Microbiol.* 2001;39:2206–2212.

[150] Hamer, D. H. Treatment of nosocomial pneumonia and trache-obronchitiscaused by multidrug-resistant *Pseudomonas aeruginosa* with aerosolized colistin. *Am. J. Respir. Crit. Care Med.* 2000;162:328–330. Brown, R. B., Kruse, J. A., Counts, G. W., Russell, J. A., Christou, N. V., Sands, M. L., Endotracheal Tobramycin Study Group. Double-blind study of endotracheal tobramycin in the treatment of gram-negative bacterial pneumonia. *Antimicrob. Agents Chemother.* 1990;34:269–272.

[151] Chapman, T. M., Perry, C. M. Cefepime: a review of its use in the management of hospitalized patients with pneumonia. *Am. J. Respir. Med.* 2003;2:75–107.

[152] Rubinstein, E., Cammarata, S., Oliphant, T., Wunderink, R., Linezolid Nosocomial Pneumonia Study Group. Linezolid (PNU-100766) versus vancomycin in the treatment of hospitalized patients with nosocomial.

[153] Wunderink, R. G., Cammarata, S. K., Oliphant, T. H., Kollef, M. H. Continuation of a randomized, double-blind, multicenter study of linezolid versus vancomycin in the treatment of patients with nosocomial pneumonia. *Clin. Ther.* 2003;25:980–992.

[154] Kollef, M. H., Ward, S., Sherman, G., Prentice, D., Schaiff, R., Huey, W., Fraser, V. J. Inadequate treatment of nosocomial infections is associated with certain empiric antibiotic choices. *Crit. Care Med.* 2000; 28:3456–3464.

[155] Gruson, D., Hilbert, G., Vargas, F., Valentino, R., Bui, N., Pereyre, S., Bebear, C., Bebear, C. M., Gbikpi-Benissan, G. Strategy of antibiotic rotation: long-term effect on incidence and susceptibilities of gram-negative bacilli responsible for ventilator-associated pneumonia. *Crit. Care Med.* 2003;31:1908–1914.

[156] Saint, S., Chenowith, C. E. Biofilms and catheter-associated urinary tract infections. *Infect. Dis. Clin. North Am.* 2003;17:411-432.

[157] Weinstein, J. W., Mazon, D., Pantelick, E., Reagan-Cirincione, P., Dembry, L. M., Hierholzer, W. J. A decade of prevalence surveys in a tertiary-care center: trends in nosocomial infection rates, device utilization, and patient acuity. *Infect. Control Hosp. Epidemiol.* 1999; 20:543-548.

[158] Strategies to prevent catheter-associated urinary tract infections in acute care hospitals. Lo, E., Nicolle, L., Classen, D., Arias, K. M., Podgorny, K., Anderson, D. J., Burstin, H., Calfee, D. P., Coffin, S. E., Dubberke, E. R., Fraser, V., Gerding, D. N., Griffin, F. A., Gross, P., Kaye, K. S., Klompas, M., Marschall, J., Mermel, L. A., Pegues, D. A., Perl, T. M., Saint, S., Salgado, C. D., Weinstein, R. A., Wise, R., Yokoe, D. S. *Infect. Control Hosp. Epidemiol.* 2008 Oct.; 29 Suppl. 1:S41-50.

[159] Tambyah, P. A., Maki, D. G. Catheter-associated urinary tract infection is rarely symptomatic. *Arch. Intern. Med.* 2000;160:678-687.

[160] Saint, S., Kaufman, S. R., Rogers, M. A. M., Baker, P. D., Boyko, E. J., Lipsky, B. Risk factors for nosocomial urinary tract related bacteremia: a case-control study. *Am. J. Infect. Control* 2006;34:401-407.

[161] Wald, H. L., Ma, A., Bratzler, D. W., et al.: Indwelling urinary catheter use in the postoperative period: Analysis of the national surgical infection prevention project data. *Arch. Surg.* 2008; 143:551–557.

[162] Willson, M., Wilde, M., Webb, M. L., et al.: Nursing interventions to reduce the risk of catheter-associated urinary tract infection: Part 2: Staff education, monitoring, and care techniques. *J. Wound Ostomy Continence Nurs.* 2009; 36:137–154.

[163] Garibaldi, R. A., Burke, J. P., Dickman, M. L., et al.: Factors predisposing to bacteriuria during indwelling urethral catheterization. *N. Engl. J. Med.* 1974; 291:215–219.

[164] Gillespie, W. A., Lennon, G. G., Linton, K. B., et al.: Prevention of urinary infection in gynaecology. *BMJ* 1964; 2:423–425.

[165] Kunin, C. M.: *Detection, prevention, and management of urinary tract infections*. Third Editon. Philadelphia, PA, Lea and Febiger, 1979.

[166] Gould, C., Umscheid, C., Agarwal, R., et al.: Guideline for Prevention of Catheter-associated Urinary Tract Infections. 2009. Available at: http:// www.cdc.gov/ hicpac/pdf/CAUTI/CAUTIguideline2009final.pdf. Accessed March 4, 2010.

[167] Warren, J. W., Platt, R., Thomas, R. J., et al.: Antibiotic irrigation and catheter-associated urinary-tract infections. *N. Engl. J. Med.* 1978; 299: 570–573.

[168] Wong, E., Hooton, T., *Centers for Disease Control: Guideline for prevention of catheter-associated urinary tract infections*. 1981. Available at: http://www.cdc.gov/ ncidod/dhqp/gl_catheter_assoc.html. Accessed March 20, 2008.

[169] Tsuchida, T., Makimoto, K., Ohsako, S., et al.: Relationship between catheter care and catheter-associated urinary tract infection at Japanese general hospitals: A prospective observational study. *Int. J. Nurs. Stud.* 2008; 45:352–361.

[170] Dieckhaus, K. D., Garibaldi, R. A.: Prevention of catheter-associated urinary tract infections. In: *Saunders infection control reference service*. Abrutytn, E., Goldmann, D. A., Scheckler, W. E. (Eds). Philadelphia, PA, WB Saunders, 1998, pp. 169–174.

[171] Wip, C., Napolitano, L.: Bundles to prevent ventilator-associated pneumonia: how valuable are they? *Curr. Opin. Infect. Dis.* 2009; 22: 159–166.

[172] Ward, V., Wilson, J., Taylor, L., et al.: *Preventing hospital-acquired infection: Clinical guidelines*. London, UK, Public Health Laboratory Service, 1997.

[173] Garnacho-Montero, J., Aldabó-Pallás, T., Palomar-Martínez, M., et al.: Risk factors and prognosis of catheter-related bloodstream infection in critically ill patients: A multicenter study. *Intensive Care Med.* 2008; 34: 2185–2193.

[174] Cruse, P. Wound infection surveillance. *Rev. Infect. Dis.* 1981; 3: 734-737.

[175] Anderson, D. J., Kaye, K. S., Classen, D., Arias, K. M., Podgorny, K., Burstin, H., Calfee, D. P., Coffin, S. E., Dubberke, E. R., Fraser, V., Gerding, D. N., Griffin, F. A., Gross, P., Klompas, M., Lo, E., Marschall, J., Mermel, L. A., Nicolle, L., Pegues, D. A., Perl, T. M., Saint, S., Salgado, C. D., Weinstein, R. A., Wise, R., Yokoe, D. S. Strategies to prevent surgical site infections in acute care hospitals., Engemann, J. J., Carmeli, Y., Cosgrove, S. E., et al. Adverse clinical and economic outcomes

attributable to methicillin resistance among patients with *Staphylococcus aureus* surgical site infection. *Clin. Infect. Dis.* 2003; 36:592-598.

[176] Kirkland, K. B., Briggs, J. P., Trivette, S. L., Wilkinson, W. E., Sexton, D. J. The impact of surgical-site infections in the 1990s: attributable mortality, excess length of hospitalization, and extra costs. *Infect. Control Hosp. Epidemiol.* 1999; 20:725-730.

[177] *Infect. Control Hosp. Epidemiol.* 2008 Oct.; 29 Suppl. 1:S51-61.

[178] Wong, E. S. Surgical site infections. In: Mayhall, C. G., ed. *Hospital Epidemiology and Infection Control.* 3rd ed. Baltimore: Lippincott, Williams, and Wilkins; 2004:287–310.

[179] Coello, R., Glenister, H., Fereres, J., et al. The cost of infection in surgical patients: a case-control study. *J. Hosp. Infect.* 1993; 25:239-250.

[180] Boyce, J. M., Potter-Bynoe, G., Dziobek, L. Hospital reimbursement patterns among patients with surgical wound infections following open heart surgery. *Infect. Control Hosp. Epidemiol.* 1990;11:89-93.

[181] Vegas, A. A., Jodra, V. M., Garcia, M. L. Nosocomial infection in surgery wards: a controlled study of increased duration of hospital stays and direct cost of hospitalization. *Eur. J. Epidemiol.* 1993;9:504-510.

[182] VandenBergh, M. F., Kluytmans, J. A., van Hout, B. A., et al. Cost- effectiveness of perioperative mupirocin nasal ointment in cardio-thoracic surgery. *Infect. Control Hosp. Epidemiol.* 1996;17:786-792.

[183] Hollenbeak, C. S., Murphy, D. M., Koenig, S., Woodward, R. S., Dunagan, W. C., Fraser, V. J. The clinical and economic impact of deep chest surgical site infections following coronary artery bypass graft surgery. *Chest* 2000;118:397-402.

[184] Whitehouse, J. D., Friedman, N. D., Kirkland, K. B., Richardson, W. J., Sexton, D. J. The impact of surgical-site infections following orthopedic surgery at a community hospital and a university hospital: adverse quality of life, excess length of stay, and extra cost. *Infect. Control Hosp. Epidemiol.* 2002;23:183-189.

[185] Apisarnthanarak, A., Jones, M., Waterman, B. M., Carroll, C. M., Bernardi, R., Fraser, V. J. Risk factors for spinal surgical-site infections in a community hospital: a case-control study. *Infect. Control Hosp. Epidemiol.* 2003;24:31-36.

[186] Horan, T. C., Gaynes, R. P., Martone, W. J., Jarvis, W. R., Emori, T. G. CDC definitions of nosocomial surgical site infections, 1992: a modification of CDC definitions of surgical wound infections. *Infect. Control Hosp. Epidemiol.* 1992;13:606-608.

[187] National Healthcare Safety Network (NHSN) members page. Available at: http://www.cdc.gov/ncidod/dhqp/nhsn_members.html. Accessed August 5, 2008.

[188] Condon, R. E., Schulte, W. J., Malangoni, M. A., Anderson-Teschendorf, M. J. Effectiveness of a surgical wound surveillance program. *Arch. Surg.* 1983;118:303-307.

[189] Kerstein, M., Flower, M., Harkavy, L. M., Gross, P. A. Surveillance for postoperative wound infections: practical aspects. *Am. Surg.* 1978;44: 210-214.

[190] Mead, P. B., Pories, S. E., Hall, P., Vacek, P. M., Davis, J. H. Jr, Gamelli, R. L. Decreasing the incidence of surgical wound infections: validation of a surveillance-notification program. *Arch. Surg.* 1986;121: 458-461.

[191] Mead, P. B., Pories, S. E., Hall, P., Vacek, P. M., Davis, J. H. Jr, Gamelli, R. L. Decreasing the incidence of surgical wound infections: validation of a surveillance-notification program. *Arch. Surg.* 1986;121: 458-461.

[192] Baker, C., Luce, J., Chenoweth, C., Friedman, C. Comparison of case-finding methodologies for endometritis after cesarean section. *Am. J. Infect. Control* 1995; 23:27-33.
[193] Cardo, D. M., Falk, P. S., Mayhall, C. G. Validation of surgical wound surveillance. *Infect. Control Hosp. Epidemiol.* 1993;14:211-215.
[194] Bratzler, D. W., Houck, P. M. Antimicrobial prophylaxis for surgery: an advisory statement from the National Surgical Infection Prevention Project. *Clin. Infect. Dis.* 2004;38:1706-1715.
[195] Bratzler, D. W., Hunt, D. R. The surgical infection prevention and surgical care improvement projects: national initiatives to improve outcomes for patients having surgery. *Clin. Infect. Dis.* 2006;43: 322-330.
[196] David, J. Riddle, Erik R. Dubberke, *Clostridium difficile* Infection in the Intensive Care Unit *Infect. Dis. Clin. North Am.* 2009 September; 23(3): 727–743.
[197] Liolios, A., Oropello, J. M., Benjamin, E. Gastrointestinal complications in the intensive care unit. *Clin. Chest Med.* 1999;20:329–345. viii.
[198] Bartlett, J. G., Chang, T. W., Gurwith, M., et al. Antibiotic-associated pseudomembranous colitis due to toxin-producing clostridia. *N. Engl. J. Med.* 1978;298:531–534.
[199] Labbe, A. C., Poirier, L., Maccannell, D., et al. Clostridium difficile infections in a Canadian tertiary care hospital before and during a regional epidemic associated with the BI/NAP1/027 strain. *Antimicrob. Agents Chemother.* 2008;52:3180–3187.
[200] Dubberke, E. R., Reske, K. A., Yan, Y., et al. Clostridium difficile--associated disease in a setting of endemicity: identification of novel risk factors. *Clin. Infect. Dis.* 2007;45:1543–1549.
[201] Bignardi, G. E. Risk factors for Clostridium difficile infection. *J. Hosp. Infect.* 1998;40:1–15.
[202] Kim, K. H., Fekety, R., Batts, D. H., Brown, D., Cudmore, M., Silva, J. Jr, Waters, D. Isolation of *Clostridiumdifficile* from the environment and contacts of patients with antibiotic-associated colitis. *J. Infect. Dis.* 1981;143(1):42-50.
[203] Fekety, R., Kim, K. H., Brown, D., Batts, D. H., Cudmore, M., Silva, J. Jr. Epidemiology of antibiotic-associated colitis; isolation of *Clostridium difficile* from the hospital environment. *Am. J. Med.* 1981;70(4):906-908.
[204] Guide to Preventing*Clostridium difficile* Infections, APIC 2013, Public Domain @ http://apic.org/Resource_/EliminationGuideForm/59397fc6-3f90-43d1-9325-e8be75d86888/File/2013CDiffFinal.pdf.
[205] Gerding, D. N., Johnson, S., Peterson, L. R., Mulligan, M. E., Silva, J. Jr. *Clostridium difficile*-associated diarrhea and colitis. *Infect. Control Hosp. Epidemiol.* 1995;16(8):459-477.
[206] Kyne, L., Hamel, M. B., Polavaram, R., Kelly, C. P. Healthcare costs and mortality associated with nosocomial diarrhea due to *Clostridium difficile*. *Clin. Infect. Dis.* 2002;34(3):346-353.
[207] Brooks, S. E., Veal, R. O., Kramer, M., Dore, L., Schupf, N., Adachi, M. Reduction in the incidence of *Clostridium difficile*-associated diarrhea in an acute care hospital and a skilled nursing facility following replacement of electronic thermometers with single-use disposables. *Infect. Control Hosp. Epidemiol.* 1992;13(2):98-103.

[208] Johnson, S., Gerding, D. N., Olson, M. M., Weiler, M. D., Hughes, R. A., Clabots, C. R., et al. Prospective, controlledstudy of vinyl glove use to interrupt *Clostridium difficile* nosocomial transmission. *Am. J. Med.* 1990 Feb.;88 (2):137-140.

[209] Riggs, M. M., Sethi, A. K., Zabarsky, T. F., Eckstein, E. C., Jump, R. L., Donskey, C. J. Asymptomatic carriers are a potential source for transmission of epidemic and nonepidemic *Clostridium difficile* strains among long-term care facility residents. *Clin. Infect. Dis.* 2007;45(8): 992-998.

[210] Badr, R. I., Badr, H. I., Ali, M. N. Mobile Phones and Nosocomial Infections. *Int. J. Infect. Control* 2012;8(2):1-5.

[211] CDC cdc,gov: http://www.cdc.gov/hai/burden.html.

[212] CDC: cdc.gov http://www.cdc.gov/drugresistance/index.html.

In: Sepsis
Editor: Nancy Khardori

ISBN: 978-1-63117-244-1

Chapter 7

Medical Device Infections and Sepsis

Lokesh Shahani, M.D.[*1] ***and Rabih O. Darouiche, M.D.***[1,2,3,4]
[1]Department of Medicine, Baylor College of Medicine, Houston, TX, US
[2]Department of Surgery, Baylor College of Medicine, Houston, TX, US
[3]Department of PM&R, Baylor College of Medicine, Houston, TX, US
[4]Michael E. DeBakey VA Medical Center, Baylor College of Medicine, Houston, TX, US

Abstract

Sepsis in simple terms is described as systemic inflammatory response to an infection. With advanced medical technology and increased longevity of the general population the use of medical devices has increased. Medical device location and application may differ widely, however all of them attract microorganisms, thus increasing the risk of infection. In this review, we focus on infections related to medical devices which are commonly used in critically and chronically ill patients.

Introduction

Sepsis is one of the oldest syndromes in medicine. Sepsis was first defined by Hippocrates as the process by which flesh rots, swamps generate foul airs, and wounds fester [1]. With the confirmation of germ theory, sepsis was redefined as a systemic infection and assumed to be the result of the host's invasion by pathogenic organisms that then spread to the bloodstream. With more understanding of the syndrome, in 1992, an international consensus panel defined sepsis as a systemic inflammatory response to infection [2]. The burden of sepsis on our health care system is significant, with approximately 750,000 cases per year in the United States, 215,000 resultant deaths, and annual costs of $16.7 billion nationally [3].

* Corresponding author: Section of Infectious Diseases, Baylor College of Medicine, 1 Baylor Plaza, Houston, TX 77030, E-mail address: lokesh83@hotmail.com

With advanced medical technology and increased longevity of the general population the use of medical devices has increased. With increased longevity there is irreparable damage to the human body resulting in functional loss or reduced quality of life. Frequently, functional restoration is achieved surgically using permanently implanted biomaterials and devices. Medical device location and application may differ widely, however all of them attract microorganisms, thus increasing the risk of infection. Continued microbial presence interferes with the intended function of an implant or device and increases the risk of infection and sepsis. In this review, we focus on infections of medical devices which are commonly used in critically and chronically ill patients as well as medical devices associated with severe infections.

Indwelling Central Venous Catheter Related Infection

Indwelling central venous catheters (CVCs) have become integral and essential to the management of diverse illnesses in and out of the hospital. They provide secure access to the central circulation for infusion therapy, nutritional support, hemodynamic monitoring, plasmapheresis and hemodialysis. In 2009, the Centers for Disease Control and Prevention (CDC) reported an estimated 23,000 episodes of central line–associated BSI (CLABSI) in American ICUs with a mortality of 12% to 25% [4].

There are 3 basic types of catheter-related "infection"—catheter colonization, catheter related blood stream infection (CLABSI), and exit-site infection [5]. Catheter colonization is the isolation of an organism from a catheter using quantitative or semi quantitative culture techniques. CLABSI is the isolation of the same organism from the bloodstream and the catheter without another source of infection. In addition, the patient must have signs or symptoms of infection, such as fever and leukocytosis. Exit-site infections involve the surrounding skin with erythema, pain, induration, and/or purulent drainage within 2 cm of the exit site of the catheter.

The Infectious Disease Society of America recommends using 1 of 3 methods to diagnose CLABSI: direct catheter culture, simultaneous blood cultures from the catheter and a peripheral site, and differential time to positivity [6]. For direct catheter culture, 15 or greater colony-forming units using semi quantitative techniques or one hundred or greater colony-forming units using quantitative techniques means the catheter is likely infected rather than colonized. Using the simultaneous culture method, if the sample from the catheter has 5 times more colony-forming units by quantitative techniques than the peripheral sample, then the catheter is likely the source. Another way to determine whether the catheter is the likely source of infection is differential time to positivity. Specimens from peripheral blood and the catheter are collected simultaneously. If the catheter specimen shows positive growth 120 minutes sooner than peripheral blood, then it is likely CLBBSI with a sensitivity of 89% and a specificity of 72% [7]. If the catheter is removed because of CLABSI, the catheter tip should be cultured. Quantitative sonication technique (>102 colony forming units [cfu] per catheter segment) and semiquantitative roll-plating method (>15 cfu per catheter segment) can be performed to aid in the diagnosis.

Catheters can be infected intraluminally (catheter hub or intravenous solution contamination), extraluminally (transversion of organisms from the skin to the intracutaneous tract), or hematogenously (distant source). The intracutaneous tract becomes contaminated at the time of catheter insertion or within the first week. In patients with short-term CVCs, extraluminal acquisition occurs, followed by the release of microorganisms from the biofilm on the implanted portion of the catheter. However, catheters placed for longer periods (>10 days) are more likely to undergo hub manipulation, which can lead to bacterial contamination followed by intraluminal colonization, resulting in blood stream infection [8].

SCOPE (Surveillance and Control of Pathogens of Epidemiological Importance), a nationwide surveillance study of nosocomial bloodstream infections in the U.S estimated a significant variation in the microbiology of the CVC related infections [9]. Coagulase negative Staphylococci (CONS) accounted for the majority i.e., 31% of the infections followed by gram negative bacilli (22%), Staphylococcus aureus (20%), Enterococcus spp. (9%) and Candida spp. (9%). Similarly according to the "US National Nosocomial Infections Surveillance System Report", the pathogens most frequently associated with CVC infections from 1991-1999 were: CONS (37%), Staphylococcus aureus (13%), Enterococcus spp. (13%), and Candida albicans (8%) [10]. Both these large studies found CONS to be the predominant organism in the 1990s.

The Healthcare Infection Control Practices Advisory Committee has published guidelines for prevention of CLABSI [11]. The key updates are listed below.

- Use ultrasound guidance to place central venous catheters to reduce the number of cannulation attempts and mechanical complications.
- Prepare clean skin with a >0.5% chlorhexidine preparation with alcohol before central venous catheter and peripheral arterial catheter insertion and during dressing changes.
- Use a chlorhexidine-impregnated sponge dressing for temporary short-term catheters in patients older than 2 months of age if the CLABSI rate is not decreasing despite adherence to basic prevention measures, including education and training, appropriate use of chlorhexidine for skin antisepsis, and maximal sterile barrier precautions.
- Use a 2% chlorhexidine wash for daily skin cleansing to reduce CLABSI.
- Use a sutureless securement device to reduce the risk of infection for intravascular catheters
- Use prophylactic antimicrobial lock solution in patients with long-term catheters who have a history of multiple CLABSI despite optimal maximal adherence to aseptic technique.
- Use a chlorhexidine/silver sulfadiazine-impregnated or minocycline/ rifampin-impregnated CVC in patients whose catheter is expected to remain in place >5 days if, after successful implementation of a comprehensive strategy to reduce rates of CLABSI, the CLABSI rate is not decreasing. The comprehensive strategy should include at least the following 3 components: educating persons, who insert and maintain catheters, use of maximal sterile barrier precautions, and a >0.5% chlorhexidine preparation with alcohol for skin antisepsis during CVC insertion.

- Use a needleless system to access IV tubing. When needleless systems are used, a split septum valve may be preferred over some mechanical valves, due to increased risk of infection with the mechanical valves.
- Use hospital-specific or collaborative-based performance improvement initiatives in which multifaceted strategies are "bundled" together to improve compliance with evidence-based recommended practices.

In patients with suspected CLABSI, empiric antibiotic therapy should be started after obtaining blood cultures. Empiric vancomycin is appropriate in most cases. Vancomycin should be replaced by beta-lactam antibiotics, for achieving better efficacy, in patients infected by methicillin-sensitive S. aureus. Daptomycin can be used as an alternative agent in institutions in which MRSA has an increased minimum inhibitory concentration (MIC) of vancomycin greater than 2 mg/mL. Coverage for MDR gram-negative organisms is recommended in severely ill patients, neutropenic patients, and those with a history of colonization by these organisms. Subsequent antibiotics are prescribed according to the identification and sensitivities of the isolate [12].

IDSA guidelines for long-term catheter-related infections recommend 4–6 weeks of antimicrobial therapy for uncomplicated S. aureus catheter related bacteremia(CRB), 7–14 days for CRB with Gram-negative bacilli or enterococcus, and a minimum of 14 days for CRB with Candida species. Complicated CRB characterized by the presence of septic thrombophlebitis and/or endocarditis should be treated for 4–6 weeks, whereas osteomyelitis should be treated for a minimum of 6–8 weeks [12].

Catheter removal with delayed CVC replacement is required in clinically unstable patients, when a persistent fever is present after 48 h, when a tunnel infection is present, or if a metastatic infectious complication are present. In clinically stable patients, in addition to systemic antibiotic therapy, the strategies for CVC management that have been studied include catheter salvage without antibiotic lock, catheter removal with delayed replacement, catheter exchange over wire, or catheter salvage with antibiotic lock. The latter three strategies address the removal or eradication of microorganisms embedded in the catheter biofilm. In general, although CVC salvage has been attempted with some success, it is more often associated with high failure rates and should be avoided [13].

Urinary Catheter Associated Infections

The urinary catheter is one of the most common invasive devices used in health care. From 12% to 16% of acute-care inpatients have an indwelling urethral catheter inserted at some time during hospitalization, including most patients admitted to critical care units [14]. Urinary infection is catheter acquired if it develops while a urinary catheter is in situ or within 72 hours after device removal. Catheter-associated bacteriuria is defined as the presence of $\geq 10^5$ colony-forming units per milliliter (cfu/ml) of one or more bacterial species in a single catheter urine specimen, and is detected in most patients who have been catheterized for >1 week. In patients with indwelling trans urethral or suprapubic catheters and in those who practice intermittent bladder catheterization, catheter associated urinary tract infection

(CAUTI) is defined as the presence of significant bacteriuria as well as the clinical symptoms and signs of UTI in the absence of other identifiable sources of infection [15].

Use of indwelling urinary catheters is increasing in long term care facilities (LTCFs). A recent survey indicated approximately 12.6% of residents newly admitted to a LTCF were found to have an indwelling urinary catheter [18]. Symptomatic UTI is the second most common infectious complication encountered in LTCFs and CAUTI is the most common cause of bacteremia and sepsis in LTCFs [19]. Diagnosis of CAUTI in LTCFs could be challenging and hence the National Healthcare Safety Network has proposed definitions for catheter-acquired urinary infection in patients with short- or long-term catheters. The proposed definition are summarized below

- At least one of the following signs or symptoms with no other recognized cause: fever (>38 C), suprapubic tenderness, costovertebral angle pain or tenderness
  or
- For patient < 1 year of age, one of fever (>38 C core), hypothermia (<36 C core), apnea, bradycardia, dysuria, lethargy, or vomiting
  and
- Urine culture with > 10^5 cfu/mL with no more than two species of microorganisms
  or
- Urine culture with >10^3 and <10^5 cfu/mL with no more than two species and positive urinalysis

A urethral catheter facilitates entry of bacteria or yeast into the bladder through several mechanisms. The most common route is extension of bacterial biofilm along the tubing and catheter, with acquisition of bladder bacteriuria correlated with duration of catheterization. In addition, periurethral organisms may be inoculated into the bladder at catheter insertion and, if the organism persists, bacteruria is established. When an indwelling catheter is not managed appropriately, contaminated urine from the drainage bag or tubing may reflux into the bladder, or organisms may be introduced when there are breaks in the closed drainage system. The bulb of the indwelling catheter prevents complete bladder drainage, and a residual pool of undrained urine remains in the bladder. Organisms, once introduced, persist in this pool of urine, and in the biofilm on the catheter or the bladder wall [16].

The initial infection after insertion of a short-term catheter is usually with a single organism, most often E coli or other Enterobacteriaceae [16]. When there is a chronic indwelling catheter, on average of three to five organisms can be isolated from the urine, including a wide variety of Enterobacteriaceae and other gram-negative organisms, gram-positive organisms, and yeast. Urease-producing organisms, such as P mirabilis, Klebsiella pneumoniae, Morganella morganii, and P stuartii, are common [17]. Candida albicans is the most common yeast, but C glabrata, C tropicalis, and others also occur. Gram-positive organisms, such as coagulase-negative staphylococci and enterococcus species, are isolated frequently, but are less likely to be associated with symptomatic infection. Bacterial isolates from patients with catheter-acquired urinary infection are characterized by increased antimicrobial resistance. This is mainly attributed to prior healthcare exposures, including repeated antimicrobial courses for urinary tract or other infections [16].

Antibiotic treatment of asymptomatic catheter-acquired urinary tract infection is not recommended because morbidity is not improved, whereas resistant organisms consistently emerge in subsequent infections. A clinical trial in critical care unit patients reported that treatment of asymptomatic bacteriuria and catheter replacement compared with no intervention was not associated with any improved patient outcomes [21].

Antimicrobial treatment of symptomatic infection must consider the known or presumed susceptibility of infecting organisms, clinical presentation, patient tolerance and renal function. The antimicrobial selected should have substantial urinary excretion, achieving high urinary levels. Current guidelines recommend that therapy for CAUTI be given for at least 7 days to limit emergence of resistant organisms [15].

The preeminent strategy to limit catheter-acquired urinary tract infection is to minimize indwelling catheter use. An indwelling urinary catheter should be inserted only for approved indications listed below and removed as soon as feasible.

- Acute urinary retention or bladder outlet obstruction
- Accurate measurement of urine output in critically ill patients
- Selected short term perioperative use
- Assist in healing open sacral or perineal wounds for incontinent patients
- Prolonged immobilization for spine or pelvic fractures
- Comfort for end-of-life care

If indwelling urinary catheter is indicated, the following practices for catheter insertion and maintenance are recommended [16]:

Catheter Insertion

- Properly trained personnel
- Hand hygiene
- Smallest-bore catheter
- Aseptic technique and sterile equipment

Catheter Maintenance

- Sterile, continuously closed drainage system
- Maintain unobstructed urine flow from bladder to drainage bag
- Standard precautions for catheter and collecting system manipulation

A multitude of novel methods for prevention of CAUTI have been developed over the past years. Ones that are routinely recommended include the use of a secured, closed, silicone urinary catheter drainage system. More recent research has focused on modification of the catheter surface by either coating or impregnation with antimicrobials or antiseptics have shown benefit in preventing UTI, however its influence on antimicrobial resistance is not known.

Ventilator Associated Infection

Ventilator associated pneumonia (VAP) is the most common nosocomial infection in critically ill patients receiving mechanical ventilation. Its reported incidence depends on the patient population, duration of mechanical ventilation, and the diagnostic criteria used. It occurs in 9-27% of mechanically ventilated patients, with about five cases per 1000 ventilator days [22]. Ventilator associated pneumonia is a type of hospital acquired pneumonia that occurs 48 hours or more are tracheal intubation [23]. It can be classified as early onset or late onset pneumonia. Early onset pneumonia occurs within four days of intubation and mechanical ventilation, and it is generally caused by antibiotic sensitive bacteria. Late onset pneumonia develops after four days and is commonly caused by multidrug resistant pathogens. Critical illness is associated with immunosuppression, and this increases susceptibility to nosocomial infections. Neutrophils are central to the body's response to most bacterial infections, and mechanically ventilated patients have neutrophil dysfunction and impaired phagocytosis leading to increased susceptibility to infections [24]. Making a diagnosis of VAP is challenging and The Centers for Disease Control and Prevention (CDC)/National Healthcare Safety Network (NHSN) has established a clinical definition (summarized below) [25].

- Patient has a baseline period of stability or improvement on the ventilator, defined by 2 or more calendar days of stable or decreasing FiO2 or PEEP.
- After a period of stability or improvement on the ventilator, the patient has evidence of worsening oxygenation.
- On or after calendar day 3 of mechanical ventilation and within 2 calendar days before or after the onset of worsening oxygenation, 1 of the following criteria is met:
  1 Purulent respiratory secretions (from 1 or more specimen collections)
    a Defined as secretions from the lungs, bronchi, or trachea that contain more than 25 neutrophils and less than 10 squamous epithelial cells per low-power field
    b If the laboratory reports semiquantitative results, those results must be equivalent to the quantitative thresholds presented earlier
  2 Positive culture (qualitative, semiquantitative, or quantitative) of sputum, endotracheal aspirate, bronchoalveolar lavage, lung tissue, or protected specimen brushing

The duration of mechanical ventilation before the onset of pneumonia is an important determinant of the likely pathogen. Pneumonia that occurs within four days of intubation is typically caused by antibiotic sensitive community bacteria such as Haemophilus spp, streptococci including Streptococcus pneumoniae, and methicillin sensitive Staphylococcus aureus. Later infection is more commonly caused by multidrug resistant pathogens, including Pseudomonas aeruginosa, Acinetobacter spp, and meticillin resistant S aureus. However, it is increasingly recognized that patients who have been in recent close contact with the healthcare system are more likely to develop infection with multidrug resistant organisms even within the first four days. Hospital admission for two or more days during the 90 days before the development of ventilator associated pneumonia, chronic haemodialysis, residence in a nursing home, and intravenous antibiotics or chemotherapy within the past 30 days all increase the likelihood of extremely drug resistant bacterial infections [26].

A high clinical suspicion of pneumonia should lead to the immediate administration of appropriate empirica antibiotics. Ideally, airway samples for microbiological analysis should be taken before administration of antibiotics as long as this does not seriously delay treatment because delayed or inappropriate initial antimicrobial treatment is associated with increased mortality.

Choose initial antibiotics on the basis of the results of local surveillance data and patient specific factors such as severity of illness, duration of hospital stay, and previous antibiotic exposure. The chosen drugs should have a high degree of activity against aerobic gram negative bacilli. Guidelines recommend third generation cephalosporin, a fluoroquinolone, or ertapenem for patients with early onset infections who have not previously received antibiotics and have no other risk factors for multidrug resistant pathogens. In those who have previously received antibiotics or who have other risk factors, including late onset pneumonia there should be concerns for drug resistant bacteria, particularly P aeruginosa. Acceptable treatment options include ceftazidime, ciprofloxacin, meropenem, and piperacillin-tazobactam. When meticillin resistant S aureus is a possibility, vancomycin or linezolid should be included in the antibiotic regimen [26].

Prevention of pneumonia is a vital part of the management of patients undergoing invasive mechanical ventilation. The three main ways of preventing pneumonia are to reduce colonization of the aerodigestive tract with pathogenic bacteria, prevent aspiration, and limit the duration of mechanical ventilation. Oral decontamination using antiseptics such as chlorhexidine seems to lower the risk of ventilator associated pneumonia especially when combined with thorough mechanical cleaning of the oral cavity. All patients without specific contraindications should be nursed in the semirecumbent position, with the head raised to 45°. Secretions that have pooled above the cuff of the tracheal tube can be removed by subglottic secretion drainage using specially designed tubes with a separate dorsal lumen that opens directly above the cuff. The duration of mechanical ventilation is strongly associated with the development of pneumonia. Therefore, strategies aimed at reducing the duration of tracheal intubation may reduce the incidence of pneumonia. Oversedation prolongs mechanical ventilation and should be avoided by careful assessment of sedation status and daily interruption of sedation if appropriate. Weaning protocols have also been shown to hasten discontinuation of mechanical ventilation [27].

Cardiovascular Implantable Electronic Device Associated Infections

The incidence of cardiovascular disease has had a constant rise among the United States' population and, subsequently, an increase in the number of patients undergoing placement of cardiovascular implantable electronic devices (CIEDs) to improve quality of life and survival. The American College of Cardiology and the American Heart Association (AHA) have issued guidelines with expanded indications for use of implantable cardioverter-defibrillators (ICDs) for primary prevention of sudden cardiac death and biventricular pacemakers (PPMs) for symptomatic improvement in patients with heart failure. With increasing use of CIEDs in the recent years, there has been a noted increase in the rate of associated infections. A recent study using data from the National Hospital Discharge Survey, estimated that 4.1% to 5.8% of CIEDs became infected between 2004 and 2006 [28].

Risk factors for CIED infections can be divided into two main groups, those that are patient-related and those that are procedure-dependent. Comorbid conditions such as heart failure, diabetes, renal insufficiency, and anticoagulation are significant risk factors for the development of CIED infection [29]. Patients with end-stage renal disease who undergo hemodialysis are at risk for dialysis-access–associated bloodstream infection, which can result in secondary infection of intravascular components of the cardiac device. Procedural factors include longer procedure time, operative inexperience, use of temporary pacing leads, dual- or triple-chamber devices, lack of antibiotic prophylaxis, and development of post-operative pocket hematomas [30].

Gram-positive organisms remain the predominant pathogens associated with CIED infection—specifically coagulase-negative staphylococci (CONS) or Staphylococcus aureus. A recent study examining CIED infections reported CONS in 41% of patients, S aureus in 41% of patients, and various gram-negative bacilli, fungi, and Propionibacterium acnes in the remainder [31].

Patients with cardiac device infections can be divided into two broad clinical categories. The first group has infection limited to the generator pocket site, with or without associated bacteremia. The second group has a primary endovascular infection with lead vegetations or an infection of intracardiac structures (endocarditis). Among patients who develop CIED infections, pocket infections occur more frequently than device-related endocarditis [32]. Further, in the MEDIC (Multicenter Electrophysiologic Device Infection Cohort) registry, the most important factor in distinguishing between local and systemic infections was time from implantation. While patients within 6 months since implantation more frequently presented with signs of local pocket infection, the majority of patients greater than 6 months since implantation presented with signs of systemic infection [33].

A recent scientific statement by the AHA on CIED infections and their management has provided formal guidance on the diagnosis of CIED infections [34]. For patients with suspected CIED infection, clinicians should perform two sets of blood cultures, tissue cultures from the generator pocket site, and cultures of the lead tips. Blood cultures should be repeated after device explantation to confirm clearance of bacteremia and to assist in determining duration of antimicrobial therapy. Transesophageal echocardiography (TEE) should be performed when patients are bacteremic, when endocarditis is suspected because of clinical findings, or when blood cultures are negative in the setting of recent antibiotic exposure.

Superficial or incisional wound infections that do not involve the device or the surgical pocket do not require extraction of the device. These infections can be managed with appropriate oral antibiotics with activity against Staphylococcal species. In general, foreign body infection requires removal of the entire CIED system to obtain eradication of the infection. Complete removal of all the components of the CIED including generator, suture sleeves, sutures and leads regardless of position (transvenous, epicardial or subcutaneous) in established CIED-related infections when infection is established or strongly suspected is the ideal goal in most cases. Extraction of all components of the CIED is required because the recurrence of infection is high if components are retained Erosion of any part of the CIED components implies contamination of the entire system, including the intravascular portion, and therefore necessitates removal of the entire system [34]. After extraction of an infected CIED, all patients should be assessed for whether a CIED is still necessary. Owing to a variety of factors number of patients may not require a new CIED implantation. In the setting of bacteremia, the timing of new CIED implantation depends on clearance of bacteremia after device extraction and presence of valvular vegetations. For patients with valvular vegetations and bacteremia, reimplantation of a CIED device can be performed 14 days from the time of the first negative blood culture after device extraction. Patients who have a lead vegetation or bacteremia without device-associated endocarditis can safely undergo implantation of a new CIED device when blood cultures drawn after device extraction are negative for 72 hours. In the setting of a generator pocket infection, generator erosion, or lead erosion, implantation of a new CIED can be performed when blood cultures are negative for 72 hours, provided there has been adequate debridement of the generator pocket. The importance of implantation on the contralateral side has been recommended. When implantation on the contralateral side is not possible, a transvenous lead can be tunneled to a device placed subcutaneously in the abdomen, or an epicardial system may be implanted [34].

Left Ventricular Assist Device Associated Infections

The left ventricular assist device (LVAD) is a mechanical pump that supplements the function of a damaged left ventricle to maintain appropriate blood flow among patients with end-stage heart failure. Use of LVADs was initially approved as a bridge to a transplant, with the aim of increasing patient survival until an appropriate organ became available. However, indications have since expanded to include permanent implantation as an alternative to heart transplantation. Despite advances in technology, post-implantation sepsis and device-related infections remain inherent risks related to the implantation. In the Randomized Evaluation of Mechanical Assistance for the Treatment of Congestive Heart Failure (REMATCH) trial, sepsis accounted for more than twice the number of deaths than did device failure in patients with LVAD [35].

Similar to CIED, infection can involve any portion of an LVAD, including the surgical site, driveline, pocket, and pump. Most infections involve the percutaneous driveline. Driveline infections span a large clinical spectrum from localized infection to widespread complicated disease, including bloodstream infection, endocarditis, and sepsis, and can occur early or late. The pump pocket is another potential site of infection. This pocket usually consists of a peritoneal space formed below the lateral rectus but can also be formed intraabdominally. Although a large praportion of pump pocket infections are believed to originate from a driveline source, inoculation of this site can occur during or after surgery, including secondary to surgical trauma or hematoma formation. LVAD-related endocarditis can be caused by ascending pump or driveline infections, bacteremia, fungemia, or can be secondary to other health care–associated infections [36].

A variety of host, device, and operative characteristics predispose to LVAD infection. Device-related risk factors seem to be correlated with increased size and surface area of the device, turbulence of flow, and available entry routes for organisms. Environmental and operative risk factors include duration of hospitalization and intensive care unit stay, use of indwelling lines and catheters, parenteral nutrition and possibly operation technique/ time, and perioperative antimicrobials used. In terms of patient factors, the severity of heart failure symptoms, as well as the presence of certain comorbid conditions, including diabetes, hyperglycemia, alcohol use, obesity and renal disease, have been associated with increased infection risk [36].

Similar to CIED infections, workup for LVAD infection includes culture and Gram stains of any potentially infected sites, blood cultures, and deep tissue swab or biopsy from driveline, pocket, or other potential sources where applicable or feasible. The AHA recommends ultrasonography for pocket site infections, and transesophageal echo-cardiography for endocarditis [37].

LVAD infection not only poses immediate morbidity and mortality but also affects candidacy for transplant because active infection carries significant risk in the setting of the substantial immunosuppression required after cardiac transplantation. Like many device or prosthesis infections, definitive treatment involves device removal, which is often impossible without concurrent transplantation. When an LVAD infection is suspected, initial treatment includes empiric broad-spectrum antimicrobials to include likely pathogens and later streamline therapy based on culture results. For localized driveline or surgical site infections, therapy is often initiated with gram positive (staphylococcal) coverage alone. Gram-negative coverage is added for pump pocket infections or deeper wound infections. Regardless of initial agent, relapse is common and infections frequently progress. Pump pocket infections with fluid collections require drainage, and some infections have been successfully treated with antimicrobial-impregnated beads. Antimicrobials should be used in combination with aggressive wound care and/or debridement where applicable. LVAD explantation with or without subsequent transplantation remains the definitive treatment of significant device-related infection but due to high morbidity and mortality, and the high risk of infection relapse [36].

Central Nervous System Device Infections

Hydrocephalus is a common neurosurgical disease and cerebrospinal fluid (CSF) diversion devices are essential in the management of this pathology. Ventriculostomy catheters (also known as external ventricular drains or EVDs) serve an increasingly important role in the neurosurgical intensive care unit (ICU). These temporary devices, which permit therapeutic CSF drainage while monitoring intracranial pressure, are used broadly; after closed head injuries, intracranial hemorrhage including subarachnoid hemorrhage (SAH), intracerebral hemorrhage (ICH), and intraventricular hemorrhage (IVH), or for hydrocephalus due to obstructing mass lesions. As with any device, however, EVDs carry a risk of infection, in this case ventriculomeningitis, in an often critically ill and complex patient population.

Ventriculomeningitis may result from contamination of the drain during insertion, contamination of the drain system during routine care and manipulation, colonization of the drain at the insertion site by skin flora, or infection of the drain and CSF as a result of a surgical-site infection. Skin flora is the main source for infection. Majority of CSF diversion device-related infections are caused by Staphylococcus spp. (coagulase-negative

Staphylococcus followed by Staphylococcus aureus). Gram negative bacilli (mostly Escherichia coli and Klebsiella spp.) are also responsible for quite a few infections [37].

There are four main mechanisms of infection that explain the development of this common complication after CSF diversion procedures: retrograde colonization of the catheter from the distal point of insertion, disruption of continuity in the skin or the surgical wound, haematogenous dissemination and catheter colonization during the surgical procedure. Risk factors for ventriculostomy-related infections commonly listed include [38]:

- Intraventricular hemorrhage
- Subarachnoid hemorrhage
- Depressed cranial fracture
- CSF leak from fracture or ventriculostomy site
- Neurosurgical operation
- Duration of catheterization
- Severity of underlying illness
- Systemic infection
- Frequent manipulation and sampling of drainage system
- Catheter irrigation

Diagnosis of CNS device infections can be challenging and hence a definition of hospital-acquired meningitis/ventriculitis has been proposed by the Centers for Disease Control and Prevention and the National Healthcare Safety Network [39]. The definition states patients must meet at least one of the following two criteria:

1 Patient has organisms cultured from CSF
2 Patient has at least one of the following signs or symptoms with no other recognized cause: fever (>38C), headache, stiff neck, meningeal signs, cranial nerve signs, or irritability and at least 1 of the following: (a) increased white cells, elevated protein, and/or decreased glucose in CSF; (b) organisms seen on Gram stain of CSF; (c) organisms cultured from blood; (d) positive antigen test of CSF, blood, or urine; (e) diagnostic single antibody titer (IgM) or fourfold increase in paired sera (IgG) for pathogen and if diagnosis is made antemortem, physician institutes appropriate antimicrobial therapy.

The main aims of the treatment of any external or internal CSF diversion device-related infection are: (1) the reduction in mortality and morbidity, (2) the maintenance of a functioning device when necessary, (3) the cure for infection. Early removal of the colonized device in combination with an immediate beginning of antibiotic therapy is strongly recommended. Due to the high rates of nosocomial staphylococci (both coagulase-negative and Staphylococcus aureus), vancomycin is routinely given as part of the first-line empiric regimen. Gram-negative infections are also common and adding an antipseudomonal agent to the empiric antimicrobial therapy is recommended.

Device removal although recommended, involves the need to divert CSF in order to avoid raised intracranial pressure as a result of the underlying condition. In this context, a new catheter placement under non-sterile conditions increases the risk for re-infection. Thus, delayed placement of a new CSF diversion device is recommended when possible. For EVDs, a second catheter insertion in the same place or in the contralateral hemisphere is recommended whenever necessary. For shunts, device removal must be followed by temporary EVD placement or even third ventriculostomy in non-communicating hydrocephalus [37]. According to the Infectious Disease Society of America guidelines on bacterial meningitis, shunt infections due to coagulase-negative staphylococci with normal CSF findings can be reshunted on the third day after removal as long as post removal cultures remain negative. If the infection is associated with CSF abnormalities, 7 days of antimicrobial therapy is recommended before replacing the shunt as long as repeat cultures are negative. If repeat CSF cultures are positive, antimicrobial treatment is continued until CSF cultures remain negative for 10 consecutive days before a new CSF shunt is placed. For infections with S aureus, fungi, and gram-negative pathogens, 10 to 14 days of antimicrobial therapy with negative follow up cultures is generally recommended [40].

Prosthetic Joint Infection

Although prosthetic joint implantations improve patients' quality of life, these procedures are associated with complications, and infection, although uncommon, is the most serious complication following joint prosthesis implantation. Prosthetic joint infections are generally classified according to the timing after surgery: early-onset infection occurs within 3 months after arthroplasty, delayed-onset infections within 3 to 24 months, and late-onset infections after 24 months [41].

Prosthetic joint infections occur most commonly because of contamination of the surgical wound with locally introduced microorganisms. Therefore, anything that delays wound healing increases the risk of infection. Although the risk of infection is primarily related to microbial inoculum, other factors such as the virulence of the microorganisms, patient-related factors, and procedure-related factors help determine susceptibility to infection. Prosthetic joints can also become infected via secondary spread related to bloodstream infections; the most common sources are skin and soft tissue, dental sources, and the urinary tract [42]. Important patient-related risk factors for prosthetic joint infection including a history of prior infection as well as a concurrent infection at the time of surgery. Procedure related risk factors include revision arthroplasty, extended operative duration, higher number of operating room personnel, postoperative bleeding or hematoma formation which could all lead to contamination of the surgical site [42].

Similar to many other device related infections, staphylococci (coagulase-negative staphylococci and S aureus) are the principal causative agents. Other gram-positive and gram-negative bacilli each represent about 20% to 25% of infections, and anaerobes, including Propionibacterium acnes, account for around 10% of the infections [41].

Although a gold standard to confirm prosthetic joint infection is lacking, diagnostic criteria have been proposed [43]. The presence of 1 or more of the following criteria is believed to be adequate for prosthetic joint infection diagnosis: acute inflammation on histopathologic examination of periprosthetic tissue, sinus tract communicating with the prosthesis, gross purulence in the joint space, or growth of the same microorganism from 2 or more cultures of joint aspirates or periprosthetic tissue. Patients with delayed-onset prosthetic joint infection may have evidence of loosening of the prosthesis or periosteal new bone formation on plain radiography, but these findings are neither specific nor sensitive [43]. If the diagnosis cannot be made preoperatively, the best approach is to obtain intra-operative periprosthetic tissue cultures to help establish the presence of prosthetic joint infection and to guide subsequent antimicrobial therapy. Because preceding antimicrobial therapy reduces the yield from both synovial fluid and operative cultures, antimicrobials should be stopped several days before revision arthroplasty to optimize yield in stable patients [42].

The main objectives of prosthetic joint infection treatment are to alleviate pain, to restore the function and to eradicate the infection. It is not always possible to achieve all three objectives and this reality explains why the decision is frequently so complex. Aggressive surgical approaches can lead to a higher chance of curing the infection, but carry the risk of worsening the functional results. At times due to patient co-morbidities when the patient is not a candidate for surgery, the approach commonly used is starting empiric antibiotics for an acute infection followed by long-term suppressive antimicrobials with the intent of symptom management and not microbiological cure. In these cases, it is essential that the infecting organism be susceptible to an oral agent that can be well tolerated over long periods.

For patients who are candidates for additional surgery, there are several possible approaches. The most conservative surgical approach is debridement with retention of device (DRD). Patients who have early-onset infection or acute onset of hematogenously acquired infection may undergo DRD followed by a prolonged course of antimicrobial therapy. For patients with delayed-onset infection, removal of the prosthesis is typically required. If a patient is not expected to gain significant function from replacement of the prosthesis, the prosthesis may simply be removed and may not be replaced. However, for most patients, the preferred approach is a staged replacement of the entire device, either as a single-stage exchange (SSE), whereby the whole implant (metallic prosthesis, cement, and accompanying biofilm) is replaced in a single procedure or, more commonly, as a 2-stage exchange (TSE). In TSE the prosthesis is removed and replaced temporarily with a polymethyl methacrylate spacer, often impregnated with antimicrobials. After 2 to 8 weeks, a new prosthesis is implanted. In addition to the surgical management, patients receive extended courses of antimicrobials. For individuals with infection associated with more virulent organisms (i.e., S aureus, gram-negative organisms), compromised soft tissue, or prolonged symptoms (>3 weeks), TSE provides superior outcomes compared with more conservative approaches. The disadvantages of TSE include an increased number of surgical procedures and prolonged periods of immobility. SSE may be appropriate for patients who have had prolonged symptoms but otherwise have intact soft tissue and less virulent organisms [42].

Conclusion

Medical device use continues to increase for the critically and chronically ill patients and has been helpful over the years to reduce morbidity and mortality in these populations. On the contrary, medical device when contaminated/colonized severe infections occur and their management is challenging. Given the current situation, producing new infection-resistant, antimicrobial biomaterials and coatings for implants and devices is the goal for the future.

References

[1] Majno G. The ancient riddle of sigma eta psi iota sigma (sepsis). *J Infect Dis* 1991;163:937-945.
[2] Bone RC, Sibbald WJ, Sprung CL. The ACCP-SCCM Consensus Conference on sepsis and organ failure. *Chest* 1992;101:1481-1483.
[3] Angus DC, Linde-Zwirble WT, Lidicker J, Clermont G, Carcillo J, Pinsky MR: Epidemiology of severe sepsis in the United States: Analysis of incidence, outcome, and associated costs of care. *Crit Care Med*29 :1303– 1310,2001.
[4] Centers for Disease Control and Prevention (CDC). Vital signs: central line associated blood stream infections–United States, 2001, 2008, and 2009. *MMWR Morb Mortal Wkly Rep* 2011;60:243–8.
[5] Pearson ML: Guidelines for prevention of intravascular device-related infections. Hospital Infection Control Practices Advisory Committee. *Infect Control Hosp Epidemiol* 17:438-473, 1996.
[6] Mermel LA, Farr BM, Sherertz RJ, et al: Guidelines for the management of intravascular catheter-related infections. *Clin Infect* Dis 32:1249- 1272, 2001.
[7] Safdar N, Fine JP, Maki DG: Meta-analysis: Methods for diagnosing intravascular device-related bloodstream infection. *Ann Intern Med* 142:451-466, 2005.
[8] Garland JS, Alex CP, Sevallius JM, et al. Cohort study of the pathogenesis and molecular epidemiology of catheter-related bloodstream infection in neonates with peripherally inserted central venous catheters. *Infect Control Hosp Epidemiol* 2008;29:243–9.
[9] Wisplinghoff H, Bischoff T, Tallent SM, Seifert H, Wenzel RP, Edmond MB. Nosocomial bloodstream infections in US hospitals: analysis of 24,179 cases from a prospective nationwide surveillance study. *Clin Infect Dis.* 2004;39(3):309.
[10] National Nosocomial Infections Surveillance (Nnis) System Report, Data Summary from January 1992-June 2001, issued August 2001. *American Journal Infection Control* 2000;29:404-21.
[11] O'Grady NP, Alexander M, Burns LA, et al. Guidelines for the prevention of intravascular catheter-related infections. *Clin Infect Dis* 2011;52:e162–93.
[12] Mermel LA, Allon M, Bouza E, et al. Clinical practice guidelines for the diagnosis and management of intravascular catheter-related infection: 2009 Update by the Infectious Diseases Society of America. *Clin Infect Dis* 2009;49:1–45.
[13] Lok CE, Mokrzycki MH. Prevention and management of catheter-related infection in hemodialysis patients. *Kidney Int.* 2011;79(6):587-98.
[14] Lo E, Nicolle L, Classen D, et al. Strategies to prevent catheter-associated urinary tract infections in acute care hospitals. *Infect Control Hosp Epidemiol* 2008;29: S41–50.
[15] Hooton, T. M. et al. Diagnosis, prevention, and treatment of catheter-associated urinary tract infection in adults: 2009 International Clinical Practice Guidelines from the Infectious Diseases Society of America. *Clin. Infect. Dis.* 50, 625–663 (2010).
[16] Nicolle LE. Urinary catheter-associated infections. *Infect Dis Clin North Am.* 2012;26(1):13-27.

[17] Warren JW, Tenney JH, Hoopes HM, et al. A prospective microbiologic study of bacteriuria in patients with chronic indwelling urethral catheters. *J Infect Dis* 1982;146:719–23.

[18] Rogers MA, Mody L, Kaufman SR, et al. Use of urinary collection devices in skilled nursing facilities in five states. *J Am Geriatr Soc* 2008;56(5):854–61.

[19] Muder RR, Brennen C, Wagener MM, et al. Bacteremia in a long-term-care facility: a five-year prospective study of 163 consecutive episodes. *Clin Infect Dis* 1992;14(3):647–54.

[20] Gould CV, Umscheid CA, Agarwal RK, et al. Guideline for prevention of catheter associated urinary tract infections 2009. Available at: *http://www.cdc.gov/hicpac/. Accessed October 14, 2013*

[21] Leone M, Perrin AS, Granier I, et al. A randomized trial of catheter change and short course antibiotics for asymptomatic bacteriuria in catheterized ICU patients. *Intensive Care Med* 2007;33:726–9.

[22] Klompas M. Does this patient have ventilator-associated pneumonia? *JAMA* 2007;297:1583-93.

[23] Boomer JS, To K, Chang KC, et al. Immunosuppression in patients who die of sepsis and multiple organ failure. *JAMA* 2011;306:2594-605.

[24] Magill SS, Fridkin SK. Improving surveillance definitions for ventilator-associated pneumonia in an era of public reporting and performance measurement. *Clin Infect Dis* 2012;54:378–80.

[25] Centers for Disease Control and Prevention: National Nosocomial Infections Surveillance System (NNIS). Available at: *http://www.cdc.gov/ncidod/dhqp/nnis.html. Accessed October 7, 2013.*

[26] American Thoracic Society; Infectious Diseases Society of America. Guidelines for the management of adults with hospital-acquired, ventilator-associated, and healthcare-associated pneumonia. *Am J Respir Crit Care Med* 2005;171:388-416.

[27] Hunter JD. Ventilator associated pneumonia. *BMJ*. 2012;344:e3325.

[28] Voigt A, Shalaby A, Saba S. Rising rates of cardiac rhythm management device infections in the United States: 1996 through 2003. *J Am Coll Cardiol* 2006;48(3): 590–1.

[29] Bloom H, Heeke B, Leon A, et al. Renal insufficiency and the risk of infection from pacemaker or defibrillator surgery. *Pacing Clin Electrophysiol* 2006;29(2):142–5.

[30] Nof E, Epstein LM. Complications of cardiac implants: handling device infections. *Eur Heart J*. 2013;34(3):229-36.

[31] Sohail MR, Uslan DZ, Khan AH, et al. Infective endocarditis complicating permanent pacemaker and implantable cardioverter-defibrillator infection. *Mayo Clin Proc* 2008;83(1):46–53.

[32] Gandhi T, Crawford T, Riddell J 4th. Cardiovascular implantable electronic device associated infections. *Infect Dis Clin North Am*. 2012;26(1):57-76.

[33] Greenspon AJ, Prutkin JM, Sohail MR, et al. Timing of the most recent device procedure influences the clinical outcome of lead-associated endocarditis results of the MEDIC (Multicenter Electrophysiologic Device Infection Cohort*)*. *J Am Coll Cardiol* 2012;59:681–687.

[34] Baddour LM, Epstein AE, Erickson CC, et al. Update on cardiovascular implantable electronic device infections and their management: a scientific statement from the American Heart Association. *Circulation* 2010;121(3):458–77.

[35] Rose EA, Gelijns AC, Moskowitz AJ, et al. Long-term use of a left ventricular assist device for endstage heart failure. *N. Engl. J. Med.* 2001; 345(20):1435–1443.

[36] Califano S, Pagani FD, Malani PN. Left ventricular assist device-associated infections. *Infect Dis Clin North Am.* 2012;26(1):77-87.

[37] Gutiérrez-González R, Boto GR, Pérez-Zamarrón A. Cerebrospinal fluid diversion devices and infection. A comprehensive review. *Eur J Clin Microbiol Infect Dis.* 2012;31(6):889-97.

[38] Stenehjem E, Armstrong WS. Central nervous system device infections. *Infect Dis Clin North Am.* 2012 Mar;26(1):89-110.

[39] Horan TC, Andrus M, Dudeck MA. CDC/NHSN surveillance definition of health care-associated infection and criteria for specific types of infections in the acute care setting. *Am J Infect Control* 2008;36(5): 309–32.

[40] Tunkel AR, Hartman BJ, Kaplan SL, et al. Practice guidelines for the management of bacterial meningitis. *Clin Infect Dis* 2004;39(9):1267–84.

[41] Zimmerli W, Trampuz A, Ochsner PE. Prosthetic-joint infections. *N Engl J Med* 2004;351:1645–54.

[42] Shuman EK, Urquhart A, Malani PN. Management and prevention of prosthetic joint infection. *Infect Dis Clin North Am.* 2012;26(1):29-39.

[43] Del Pozo JL, Patel R. Clinical practice. Infection associated with prosthetic joints. *N Engl J Med* 2009;361:787–94.

In: Sepsis
Editor: Nancy Khardori

ISBN: 978-1-63117-244-1

Chapter 8

Molecular Diagnostics and Inflammatory Biomarkers in Diagnosis of Sepsis

Chand Wattal*, MBBS, M.D. and Reena Raveendran, MBBS, M.D.
Dept of Clinical Microbiology and Immunology, GRIPMER,
Sir Ganga Ram Hospital, New Delhi, India

Abstract

Sepsis is a leading cause of mortality in critically ill patients. Immediate diagnosis and appropriate antibiotic initiation are essential to reduce mortality. However, differentiating sepsis from non-infectious causes of systemic inflammatory response syndrome (SIRS) is difficult, especially in critically ill patients who may have SIRS due to other causes. The most commonly studied biomarkers of sepsis are reviewed for their current uses and diagnostic accuracies along with the newer bio-markers with their potential utility. Single ideal biomarker has not yet been identified. The research focus has to shift to assessing the diagnostic relevance of combined use of multiple biomarkers.

Introduction

Sepsis is a common and serious problem in critically ill patients, both as a cause of admission to critical care units and healthcare –associated infection following admission. At present, sepsis is a leading cause of death in critically ill patients associated with a mortality rate as high as 60%, despite the use of modern antibiotics and resuscitation therapies. [1, 2] An important factor deciding the survival of these patients is an early diagnosis which increases the possibility of starting timely and appropriate treatment. [3] With accurate

* Corresponding author: chandwattal@gmail.com

diagnosis of sepsis, not only can appropriate antibiotics be administered promptly, but also can avoid unnecessary antimicrobial usage to combat escalating rates of antibiotic resistance.

A high proportion of critically ill patients have the systemic inflammatory response syndrome (SIRS). The term sepsis is applied when infection is suspected in addition to SIRS. [4] The gold standard for sepsis diagnosis has been considered to be microbial cultures. [5] However, the major limitations of culture-based technology are the time taken, and the lack of sensitivity for slow growing and non-cultivable microorganisms. In addition, many of these patients would have received recent antimicrobial therapy that can render cultures negative. Studies have reported negative culture results in as many as 30-40% of ICU patients with severe sepsis. [6] In light of these limitations, alternative diagnostic methods using biological laboratory markers (biomarkers) play an important role in the diagnosis of sepsis. These markers are more helpful in ruling out than in ruling in an infection. To be clinically useful, a sepsis biomarker needs to provide information additional to that already available from established clinical assessments. It needs to be able to differentiate bacterial infection from non-infective and viral causes of SIRS, and also be available in a timely and cost-effective manner. In addition to diagnosis of sepsis, other potential uses of biomarkers include their role in prognostication, guiding antimicrobial therapy, and evaluating the response to therapy. [7] More than 170 different compounds have been suggested as potential biomarkers of sepsis [7] but few have been studied extensively such as CRP and PCT, others have been suggested more recently and not evaluated extensively. The purpose of this chapter is to give an overview of the most commonly studied biomarkers of sepsis with relevance to the present day critical care practice.

Biomarkers in Present Use

C - Reactive Protein

C - reactive protein (CRP) is an acute-phase reactant protein produced and secreted by hepatocytes as part of an immediate response to infection or tissue injury. CRP was first described in the early 1930s, [8] and since then is being extensively investigated for its role in diagnosis of sepsis. It is a member of the pentraxin (from the Greek "penta" meaning 5 and "ragos" meaning berries) family of calcium-dependent ligand-binding plasma proteins. The pentraxin family is highly conserved in evolution, suggesting that members have an important physiologic role. The other member of this family present in humans is serum amyloid P component. The human CRP molecule is composed of 5 identical nonglycosylated polypeptide subunits, each containing 206 amino acid residues, forming an annular configuration. [9] CRP is synthesized within six to eight hours of exposure to an infective process or inflammation, with a half life of 19 hours. In healthy young adults, the normal plasma concentration of CRP is about 0.8mg/dL. [10] Its concentration in blood rises up to 1000 fold in response to inflammation and infection. [11] Even though the precise biologic properties of CRP are controversial, it has been suggested that it may act in a pro-inflammatory or in an anti-inflammatory capacity to aid host defense. In vitro, CRP has been shown to increase release of the anti-inflammatory cytokine IL-10 and decrease synthesis of several proinflammatory cytokines including IL-12, tumor necrosis factor and interferon-γ.

CRP also activates complement, enhances phagocytosis, inhibits activated neutrophils, increases nitric oxide synthesis, and induces tissue factor and adhesion molecule expressions. [12] The plasma clearance of CRP is similar in healthy individuals and in those with disease, and the synthesis rate is the only significant determinant of its plasma level, making measurement of CRP levels a useful objective index of the acute phase response [11]

Many studies have now been published that demonstrated increased CRP levels in patients with sepsis. [13, 14, 15] Studies have shown CRP to have sensitivity varying from 30 to 97.2% and specificity values varying from 75-100% for infection. [16, 17, 18, 19] In 190 adult patients in ICU, Ugarte and colleagues reported a sensitivity of 67.6% and specificity of 61.3% for diagnosis of infection using a cutoff value of 7.9mg/dL. [17] In 112 ICU patients, Povoa et al reported that a serum CRP concentration greater than 8.7mg/dL had a sensitivity of 93.4% and a specificity of 86.1% for infection and the combination of CRP >8.7 mg/dL and temperature >38.2^{0}C increased the specificity for diagnosing infection to 100%. [18] Sierra and colleagues reported a sensitivity of 94.3% and specificity of 87.3% using a cutoff of 8mg/dL. [19]

CRP is a nonspecific marker of sepsis because its blood levels are increased in other inflammatory conditions like rheumatoid arthritis, Crohn's disease, acute myocardial infarction, pancreatitis etc. [12] Because baseline CRP levels are often raised as a result of co-morbid chronic conditions, particularly in ICU patients in whom other causes of inflammation may be present, changes in concentrations over time are more useful than single values. Following the pattern of CRP levels over time may provide a clearer picture, with an increasing CRP level suggesting an infection is developing or worsening. [12] In an observational cohort study, a maximum daily CRP variation of greater than 4.1mg/dL predicted nosocomial infection with a sensitivity of 92.1% and a specificity of 71.4%; and in combination with a CRP concentration greater than 8.7mg/dL, the discriminative power increased even further to a sensitivity of 92.1% and specificity of 82.1%. [20] In a study by Lobo et al, it was concluded that CRP levels are a good early marker of morbidity and mortality in ICU patients.

The authors suggest serial measurement of CRP concentrations in critically ill patients may help identify patients who may require more aggressive diagnostic and therapeutic interventions to avoid complications. [21] It is important to note that CRP should not be used as a marker of infection in patients with fulminant liver failure, as CRP levels do not always increase in the presence of sepsis in those patients. [22]

The role of CRP in distinguishing between different types of infections like bacterial, fungal or viral is not very reliable. In general CRP concentrations are higher in bacterial infections than in other causes. A study by Martini et al in surgical ICU patients reported that CRP levels in patients with bacterial sepsis (115-316mg/dL) were higher than those in patients with candidal sepsis (66-129mg/dL). [23] Several studies have examined the diagnostic relevance of CRP in viral infections and the current data suggest that CRP is an unreliable marker for viral infections on its own. [24] It is unclear if CRP can be used to distinguish Gram-positive from Gram-negative bacterial infections. In a retrospective study of patients with nosocomial bacteremia, serum CRP levels were substantially higher in patients with gram-negative bacteremia than in those with gram-positive bacteremia. [25]

In conclusion, even though CRP is not a specific test for sepsis, its low cost, ease of use and wide availability has made CRP a popular test as a supporting evidence in patients with signs and symptoms of sepsis.

When considering the use of serum CRP levels in critically ill patients, 3 key principles should be remembered. [14]

1. CRP levels are more useful to rule out than to rule in sepsis
2. Serial measurement of CRP over time is more important than a single value.
3. Serum CRP levels should always be used in conjunction with other clinical signs and symptoms.

Procalcitonin

Procalcitonin (PCT) is the precursor protein of the hormone calcitonin. PCT is synthesized physiologically by thyroid C cells but in sepsis has an extra-thyroidal origin. PCT was first found elevated in sepsis in 1993. [26] Normal serum and plasma levels of PCT are less than 0.1ng/mL. Levels above this value have been accepted to be pathological and is synthesized in various extra thyroidal neuroendocrine tissues. [27, 28] PCT has various immunologic functions, modulating the immune response during sepsis, infection, and inflammation. Among those functions are chemotactic functions, modulation of inducible nitric oxide synthase, cytokine induction, and the protein interferes with receptor binding of other peptide hormones involved in modulating intravascular fluid and vascular tone (calcitonin gene–related peptide, adrenomedullin). Induction of the protein is strictly regulated and depends on cell-cell interactions. Circulating blood cells produce cytokines, but not PCT. Migration of adherent monocytic cells into the tissue plays a major role in PCT induction because only adherent monocytic cells produce PCT in a time-dependent manner and contact of such cells with adipocytes, for example, triggers a major and sustained PCT response in vitro. [29].

PCT differs from other proposed sepsis markers such as cytokines, C-reactive protein (CRP), or lipopolysaccharide-binding protein (LBP) primarily by the fact that it better reflects the severity of the systemic inflammatory response to infection, and it has some potential to differentiate between the infectious and sterile causes of systemic inflammation [29] PCT levels start to increase after 2 hours of an infectious stimulus and peak at between 8 and 24 h. This response is considerably faster than that of CRP, whose levels increase slowly and only peak at 36 h after an endotoxin challenge. [30, 31] The rapid up regulation and sustained PCT levels in the serum during infection make it an ideal biomarker. A PCT value of 0.25 to 0.5 ng/mL suggests the presence of a bacterial infection that requires antimicrobial treatment. If PCT levels are less than 0.25ng/mL, severe bacterial infection and sepsis are very unlikely; however, local infection may be present. [29] There have been a number of studies looking at the diagnostic ability of PCT in critically ill patients and, more specifically, its ability to differentiate between SIRS and bacterial sepsis. PCT was found to be significantly elevated in patients with sepsis, severe sepsis and septic shock. Especially high concentrations were found in patients with severe stages of the disease like severe sepsis or septic shock. [32,33,34] A meta-analysis done by Uzzan et al in 2006 reviewed and analyzed 25 studies with a total of 2966 patients where the sensitivity ranged from 42% to 100% and the specificity from 48% to 100%. A sub analysis of this meta-analysis on 15 studies to compare the diagnostic ability of PCT versus CRP showed a sensitivity and specificity for CRP ranging from 35% to 100% and from 18% to 84% respectively. [35] Uzzan et al concluded that PCT represents a good biological diagnostic marker for sepsis, severe sepsis and septic shock. Another review by Chan et al in 2011 reported sensitivity and specificity values ranging from 74.8-100% and 70-100% respectively for PCT in the diagnosis of sepsis. [16]

Because the level of PCT is related to the severity of the systemic inflammatory response, PCT values have some prognostic value as well. Studies have reported that levels of PCT are a good indicator of response to treatment, [36, 37] severities of sepsis [36] and mortality from sepsis. [36, 38] But it is unclear whether PCT can be used to distinguish between gram-positive and gram-negative bacterial infections [16, 54].

The use of PCT levels to guide antibiotic therapy has been tested in several clinical trials in different groups of infected patients. Because the negative predictive value to exclude sepsis and severe bacterial infections is high, PCT has successfully been evaluated to guide antibiotic therapy in various types of patients, such as outpatients with suspected lower respiratory tract infections (LRTIs) and critically ill patients with sepsis, severe sepsis, and septic shock. Despite reported beneficial effects on antibiotic utilization in many studies, not all support these findings. [40] PCT-guided antibiotic stewardship resulted in a reduction of antibiotic exposure between 20% and 70% without a negative effect on patient outcomes. [41] Schuetz et al reported, in a meta-analysis of 14 trials in patients with acute respiratory infection, that use of PCT to guide initiation and duration of antibiotic treatment was effective in reducing antibiotic exposure without an increase in the risk of mortality or treatment failure. [42].

Procalcitonin has also been used to distinguish fungal and viral infections from bacterial infections. During viral infections, PCT levels are reported to remain low. In a study on 122 children with viral infections, the maximum PCT level observed was 0.7ng/mL. [43] PCT was used to differentiate bacterial from viral meningitis. [36] Studies have shown that fungal infections tend to cause mild elevations in PCT concentration compared with levels seen in bacterial infections. [39, 44].

However several investigators have questioned the diagnostic and prognostic accuracy of routine PCT measurements, reporting inconsistent and variable results depending on the severity of illness and infection in the patient population studied. A Meta-analysis by Tang et al found mean values of 71% (95% CI 67-76%) for both sensitivity and specificity and an area under the receiver operating curve (AUROC) of 0.78 (95% CI 0.73-0.83). [45] As with CRP, PCT levels are raised in other inflammatory conditions including pancreatitis, acute myocardial infarction, post surgery and trauma. Given the fact that PCT can be elevated in certain non-infective conditions as well, it is probably better used to rule out than rule in bacterial infection.

Despite the limitations of PCT, to date, there is no other biomarker that differentiates better between the infectious and noninfectious causes and severity of inflammation in patients with a systemic inflammatory response. This is especially true in comparison with CRP, LBP and interleukin 6. [29]

A false-negative result can occur if samples are taken too early in the course of infection and a repeat test is advised at 6-12h. However, if all microbiologic cultures are negative and a clear source of infection has not declared itself by 24 h, a repeat low PCT, combined with clinical judgment, provides a strong argument for discontinuing antimicrobial therapy and searching for an alternative diagnosis. Such an approach is likely to avoid >3-4days of broad-spectrum antibiotic therapy. [46]

Newer Markers of Sepsis

The extensive research centered on the discovery of the ideal biomarker of sepsis which would allow for the early recognition of infection has lead to the discovery of a vast array of newer biomarkers.

Cytokine Levels

Cytokines are proteins secreted by components of the innate and adaptive immune systems, and they act as effectors or modulators of inflammatory response which in turn play an essential role as mediators of sepsis. In response to antigens such as bacterial endotoxins, activated tissue macrophages produce TNF-α and IL1. These proinflammatory cytokines in turn lead to the initiation of cytokine cascade resulting in increased production of IL6, IL8 and chemokines. Various cytokines have been assessed for their role as biomarkers of sepsis and the most important ones with promising results are IL-6, TNF and IL-8. Serum levels of cytokines have been shown to be associated with sepsis in multiple studies. [47, 48] Raised serum levels have also been shown to be associated with development of organ dysfunction and mortality. [49] In a study by Bozza et al. the prognostic value of 17 cytokines were evaluated using a multiplex analysis system in a multicenter cohort study of 60 patients. The study demonstrated distinct cytokine profiles associated with sepsis severity, evolution of organ failure and death. [48]

In a study by Mera et al, where 17 cytokines were measured, initial levels of IL-8 were shown to have the most predictive value for fatal outcome. [50] Other cytokines like IL1β, IL6, IL8, IL12, IFNγ, G-CSF and TNF-α levels were also high in non-survivors. Studies in neonates have shown that umbilical cord blood IL6 to be a sensitive marker for diagnosing early onset neonatal sepsis, with sensitivities of 87-100% and negative predictive values of 93-100%. [51, 52] Detection of IL8 levels along with CRP has been reported to enhance the diagnostic value for neonatal sepsis. [53] Despite some of the promising results with cytokines as biomarkers in sepsis, they fail to fulfill many of the tenets required of an ideal sepsis marker because of their relative insensitivity and lack of specificity. These cytokines are all involved in the inflammatory response to infection, but levels are also increased in patients with other inflammatory processes such as arthritis, post trauma and surgery and even in myocardial infarction [54].

Soluble Triggering Receptor Expressed on Myeloid Cells-1 (sTREM-1)

Recently a new family of receptors expressed on myeloid cells, the triggering receptor expressed on myeloid cells-1, has been described. It is a member of the immunoglobulin superfamily, the expression of which is up regulated in the presence of bacteria or fungi. [55, 56] At the same time TREM-1 is not up regulated in patients with noninfectious inflamematory disorders such as psoriasis, ulcerative colitis or vacuities caused by immune complexes. [55] Studies in mice have shown that the activation of TREM-1 in the presence of toll-like receptor (TLR) 2 or TLR4 ligands amplifies the production of proinflammatory cytokines (TNF-α, IL-1β, granulocyte-macrophage colony stimulating factor), together with the inhibition of IL-10 release. In addition, activation of these TLRs up regulates TREM-1expression. Thus, TREM-1 and TLRs seem to cooperate in producing an inflammatory response. [57] In addition to its membrane-bound form, a soluble form of TREM-1 is liberated by the cleavage of its extracellular domain. Soluble TREM-1 (sTREM-1) acts as a decoy receptor, sequestering TREM-1 ligand, which may exist in soluble form in the sera of septic patients, and dampen TREM-1 activation. [57]

Considering the modest reliability of traditional biomarkers, such as C-reactive protein (CRP) and PCT, and the a prior specific involvement of TREM-1 during infections, the usefulness of sTREM-1 in diagnosing sepsis has been the focus of several studies during the recent 5 years. In a study by Gibot et al., [58] the plasma concentrations of CRP, PCT and sTREM-1 were higher in infected patients than in those with noninfectious SIRS. sTREM-1 performed better than other markers in diagnosing. Infection, with sensitivity and specificity values of 96% and 89% respectively. Another study by Zhang et al also suggested that sTREM-1 is more sensitive and specific for infection than other markers including CRP and PCT. [59] But 2 subsequent studies in ICU patients by Barati et al and Gemez et al came out with not so encouraging results, in which the sensitivity ranged from 60-70% and specificity from 59-60%. [60, 61] Therefore, the measurement of plasma sTREM-1 concentrations does not seem to hold its initial promise in diagnosing systemic infections. Indeed, recent evidences suggest that many inflammatory conditions may be responsible for an elevation of plasma sTREM-1 concentrations. [57] A recent meta-analysis on the diagnostic utility of sTREM-1 in 11 studies comprising 1795 patients, showed a pooled sensitivity and specificity of 79% (95% CI 65-89%) and 80% (95% CI 69-88%), respectively, with an area under the ROC curve of 0.87 (95% CI 0.84-0.89). The authors concluded that plasma sTREM-1 was inadequate as a single biomarker for diagnosing sepsis. Whether this marker can predict sepsis in association with other markers warrants additional studies.

Cell Surface Markers

Various neutrophil as well as lymphocyte surface markers have been under evaluation for their utility as sepsis biomarkers. It is believed that assessing the cellular response to cytokines may be a better way of evaluating early immunologic response to bacterial invasion. Also advances in flow cytometry technology have opened up ways of detecting the activated cell surface markers with considerable efficiency. [62] Currently, neutrophil surface marker CD64 is the most evaluated cell surface marker. The expression of CD64 on the neutrophil membrane is negligible in health, but up regulated in response to proinflammatory cytokines as in sepsis and other inflammatory conditions such as arthritis. Neutrophil CD64 expression has been reported to have variable sensitivity and specificity for sepsis diagnosis and prognosis. [54] In a study of 132 emergency department patients with fever, 87% of whom had bacterial infection, the CD64 index was higher in patients with infection than in those without (3.7 ± 3.2 vs 2.5 ± 2.3; p = 0.03); the AUROC for detection of bacterial infection was 0.66 (95% CI: 0.52–0.8) and for prediction of survival it was 0.71 (95% CI: 0.57–0.85).[63] In another study by Gros et al. on 293 ICU patients with suspected sepsis, the sensitivity and specificity of CD464 in diagnosing sepsis was reported to be 63% and 89% respectively. [48] The authors concluded that as a result of its weak sensitivity, but high specificity, the CD64 index may be useful in combination with a more sensitive biological marker. CD11b is another neutrophil surface marker, normally expressed at a very low concentration on the surface of non-activated neutrophils. There is a 2–4-fold increase in neutrophil CD11b expression in infants with blood culture positive sepsis, [60, 61] similar to that seen in adults with blood culture positive sepsis. The sensitivity and specificity of CD11b for diagnosing early onset neonatal sepsis are 86.3–100% and 100% respectively. [62] There are many other lymphocyte and neutrophil surface markers under study for their diagnostic utility in sepsis.

Serum Amyloid A

Serum amyloid A (SAA) is an apolipoprotein mainly produced by liver. They are regarded as acute-phase proteins because they increase considerably during infection. They can show as much as 1000 fold increase in 8 to 24 h after the onset of sepsis. [65] Compared with CRP, SAA is reported to rise faster and higher after the onset of sepsis and remain at higher relative elevations. Although the data about its use in diagnosis of sepsis is limited, it is reported to have potential for diagnosing sepsis. Most of the studies have evaluated its role in the diagnosis of neonatal sepsis and has been suggested to be a superior marker compared with CRP. [65,66] In a meta analysis done by Yuan et al, SAA test showed better accuracy than CRP for the diagnosis of neonatal sepsis. The authors suggest that the combination of SAA with CRP and PCT will improve the diagnosis of sepsis. [67]

The Future Sepsis Biomarkers

Sepsis biomarkers are currently more useful in ruling out a diagnosis of sepsis than to actually identify sepsis. But recent advances in molecular biology and biochemistry have lead to the discovery of potential new biomarkers for sepsis. Many of them are under standardization so that the usefulness of different markers may be analyzed. At the same time the ongoing search for an ideal biomarker for sepsis is still underway. Some of the markers recently added to the list of potential biomarkers for sepsis and are still under evaluation include the following.

Endotoxin Activity Assay

Endotoxin, an outer membrane component of gram-negative bacteria, is a well described mediator of severe sepsis. Endotoxemia has been described in sepsis caused by all pathogen classes probably as a result of endogenous release from liver and spleen because of splanchnic hypoperfusion. [68, 69] Until recently, endotoxin levels were measured using a limulus amebocyte lysate assay which is time consuming and also known for its false positive and false negative test results. A new rapid endotoxin assay (endotoxin activity assay [EAA]) is approved by the Food and Drug Administration for assessing the risk of developing severe sepsis in patients in ICU. Endotoxin activity of 0.4 is approximately equivalent to 25 to 50 pg/mL. [68] A study by Marshall et al concluded that the EAA may be a useful diagnostic tool for the investigation of invasive gram-negative infection and incipient sepsis. In 74 consecutive ICU admissions, EAA levels were higher in patients with a diagnosis of sepsis (470 ± 57 pg/mL) than in patients admitted with a diagnosis other than sepsis (157 ± 140 pg/mL; $P < 0.001$). [70]

Angiopoietin

Angiopoietin (Ang)-1 and -2 are endothelial-derived vascular growth factors that have contrasting roles in endothelial activation during sepsis. Angiopoietin-1 is a ligand for the tyrosine kinase receptor with immunoglobulin and epidermal growth factor domains (Tie2); stabilizes the endothelium, inhibiting vascular leakage and inflammatory gene expression, and prevents recruitment and transmigration of leukocytes. Angiopoietin-2 competes with Angiopoietin-1 for the Tie2 receptor which results in destabilization of the endothelium, increased capillary permeability, endothelial apoptosis, and increased expression of adhesion molecules. [68]. Numerous studies have now demonstrated increased angiopoietin-2 levels in the setting of sepsis. In a study by Siner et al, elevated circulating serum Ang-2 levels were associated with increased hospital mortality in patients with sepsis. Circulating Ang-2 levels were significantly higher ($P = 0.01$) in those who died (24.9 ng/mL; interquartile range, 21.5-38.0 ng/mL) compared with those who survived (13.5 ng/mL; interquartile range, 8.1-21.6 ng/mL). [71] In another study by Ricciuto et al describing 70 patients with severe sepsis, survivors had higher peak Ang-1 levels (median:13 vs 10 ng/mL; p=0.019) and lower Ang-2 levels (median:2.8 vs 6.2 ng/mL; p=0.013). [72]

Growth Arrest-specific Protein 6

The product of growth arrest-specific gene 6 (Gas6) is a vitamin K dependent protein that is secreted by Leucocytes and endothelial cells in response to injury and participates in cell survival, proliferation, migration and adhesion. [54, 73] In a case-controlled study by Borgel et al. Gas6 plasma levels were quantified using enzyme-linked immunosorbent assay. Gas6 plasma levels were elevated (110 [75-139] ng/mL) in severe sepsis patients compared with organ failure patients unrelated to infection (85 [56- 101] ng/mL) and healthy subjects (54 [49- 68] ng/mL). [74] In a study by Gibot et al, Gas6 protein strongly correlated with both PCT and sTREM-1 concentrations. [73] But there was no difference in Gas6 protein levels among survivors and non survivors.

Proteomics, Genomics and PCR

New proteomics, genomic and microarray techniques are being used to identify potential biomarker candidates that could be used to diagnose, guide therapy or evaluate prognosis in patients with sepsis. [54] These new technologies enable the expression of multiple proteins or genes to be evaluated simultaneously in which patterns or profiles of genes and/or protein expression are used to identify and follow sepsis. Few studies are already done substantiating the potential use of these techniques. [54]

Molecular methods based on PCR technology have also been developed to help the diagnosis of infection [54, 75] by amplifying specific regions of bacterial DNA, these PCR probes allow minute traces of DNA to be detected, providing positive results when traditional cultures are still negative. Several such tests are now commercially available (e.g.,: SeptiFast, Roche Diagnostics, Mannheim, Germany) which enable the identification of many of the most common bacterial and fungal pathogens from blood samples. In a study by Pasqualini et al, the SeptiFast assay was shown to have better specificity for pathogen identification (100 vs 94%; p=0.005) and a higher positive predictive value (100 vs 75%; p=0.005) than blood cultures. [76] Another study using a multiplex PCR, VYOO (SIRS-LAB, Jena, Germany) reported that concordance in bacterial identification between microbiology and the VYOO test was 46.2%. This study demonstrated that this new technology offers great hopes, but improvements are still needed. [77]

Conclusion

Considering the complexities of sepsis response, the different times at which individual biomarkers are elevated, and the fact that most of the biomarkers currently available are also raised in other inflammatory conditions, it is unlikely that any single 'gold standard biomarker' will ever exist for the diagnosis of sepsis. Thus the research should shift focus on to assessing the combined diagnostic capabilities of multiple biomarkers. Combination panels of biomarkers or sepsis scores are likely to replace individual biomarker levels, but the challenge is to determine which variables should be included in such scores. New technologies like proteomics, genomics and multiplex PCR will have to be studied to determine the impact of these methods on patient-based outcomes and evaluate their cost-effectiveness. The need of the day is a multiplex point of care test kit for sepsis diagnosis which would be of clinical use in rural areas and low income countries as well. Further studies are needed to determine which elements should be included in such a system. With continued advances in this field, in the not so distant future, physicians may be able to determine, the likelihood of a patient developing sepsis, the response to treatment, and the likely prognosis of patient at the point-of-care.

References

[1] Angus DC, Linde-Zwirble WT, Lidicker J, Clermont G, Carcillo J, Pinsky MR. Epidemiology of severe sepsis in the United States: analysis of incidence, outcome, and associated costs of care. *Crit Care Med.* 2001;29:1303-1310.

[2] Kauss IAM, Grion CMC, Cardoso LTQ, et al. The epidemiology of sepsis in a Brazilian teaching hospital. Brailian J. Infect. Dis. 2010;14(3):264-270.

[3] Kumar A, Roberts D, Wood K, et al. Duration of hypotension before initiation of effective antimicrobial therapy is the critical determinant of survival in human septic shick. *Crit Care Med.* 2006;34:1589-96.

[4] Definitions of sepsis and organ failure and guidelines for the use of innovative therapies in sepsis. American College of Chest Physicians/Society of Critical Care Medicine Consensus Conference. *Crit Care Med.* 1992; 20:864-874.

[5] Wang P, Yang Z, He Y, Shu C. Pitfalls in the rapid diagnosis of positive blood culture. Rev. Med. Microbiol. 2010;21(3):39-43.

[6] Vincent JL, Rello J, Sprung CL, et al. Sepsis in European intensive care units: results of the SOAP study. *Ctit. Care Med.* 2006;34(2):344-353.

[7] Pierrakos C, Vincent JL. Sepsis biomarkers: a review. Crit Care. 2010;14(1):R15.

[8] Tillett WS, Francis T. Serological reactions in pneumonia with a non-protein somatic fraction of Pneumococcus. *J. Exp. Med.* 1930.52(4):561-571.

[9] Thompson D, Pepys MB, Wood SP. The physiological structure of human C-reactive protein and its complex with phosphocholine. *Structure* 1999;7:169-77.

[10] Raitakari M, Mansikkaniemi K, Marniemi J, et al. Distribution and determinants of serum high-sensitive C-reactive protein in a population of young adults: the cardiovascular risk in young Finns study. *J. Intern Med.* 2005;258:428-34.

[11] Vigushin DM, Pepys MB, Hawkins PN. Metabolic and scintigraphic studies of radioiodinated human C-reactive protein in health and disease. *J. Clin. Invest.* 1993;91(4):1351-7.

[12] Vincent JL, Donadello K, Schmit X. Biomarkers in the critically ill patient: C-reactive protein. *Crit. Care Clin.* 2011;27(2):241-251.

[13] Povoa P, Coelho L, Almeida E, et al. C-reative protein as a marker of infection in critically ill patients. *Clin. Microbiol Infect.* 2005;11(2):101-108.

[14] Schmit X, Vincent JL. The time course of blood C-reactive protein concentrations in relation to the response to the initial antimicrobial therapy in patients with sepsis. *Infection* 2008;36:213-219.

[15] Keshet R, Boursi B, Maoz R, Shnell M, Guzner-Gur H. Diagnostic and prognostic significance of serum C-reative protein levelsin patients admitted to the department of medicine. *Am. J. Med. Sci.*2009;337(4):248-255.

[16] Chan T, Gu F. Early diagnosis of sepsis using serum biomarkers. *Expert Rev Mol Diagn.* 2011;11(5):487-496.

[17] Ugarte H, Silva E, Mercan D, et al. Procalcitonin used as a marker of infection in the intensive care unit. *Crit Care Med.*1999;27:498-504.

[18] Povoa P, Coelho L, Almeida E, et al. C-reactive protein as a marker of infection in critically ill patients. *Clin. Microbiol Infect.* 2005;11:101-8.

[19] Sierra R, Rello J, Bailen MA, et al. C-reactive protein used as an early indicator of infection in patients with systemic inflammatory response syndrome. *Intensive Care Med.* 2004;30:2038-45.

[20] Povoa P, Coelho L, Almeida E, et al. Early identification of intensive care unitacquired infections with daily monitoring of C-reactive protein: a prospective observational study. *Crit Care.* 2006;10:R63.

[21] Lobo SMA, Lobo FRM, Bota DP, Lopes-Ferreira F, Soliman HM, Mélot C, Vincent JL. C-reactive protein levels correlate with mortality and organ failure in critically ill patients. *Chest.* 2003 Jun;123(6):2043-9.

[22] Silvestre JP, Coelho LM, Povoa PM. Impact of fulminant hepatic failure in C-reactive protein? *J. Crit Care.* 2010;25(4):657.e7-12.

[23] Martini A, Gottin L, Menestrina N, et al. Procalcitonin levels in surgical patients at risk of candidemia. *J. Infect.* 2010;60:425–30.

[24] Quint JK, Donaldson GC, Goldring JJP, Baghai-Ravary R, Hurst JR, Wedzicha JA. Serum IP-10 as a biomarker of human rhinovirus infection at wxacerbation of COPD. *Chest.* 2010;137(4):812-822.

[25] Vandijck DM, Hoste EA, Blot SI, et al. Dynamics of C-reactive protein and white blood cell count in critically ill patients with nosocomial Gram positive vs. Gram-negative bacteremia: a historical cohort study. *BMC Infect Dis.* 2007;7:106.

[26] Assicot M, Gendrel D, Carsin H, et al. High serum procalcitonin concentrations in patients with sepsis and infection. *Lancet.* 1993;341:515–518.

[27] Whicher J, Bienvenu J, Monneret G. Procalcitonin as an acute phase marker. *Ann. Clin. Biochem.* 2001;38:483-493.

[28] Assicot M, Gendrel D, Carsin H, Reymond J, Guilbaud J, Bohuon C. High serum procalcitonin concentrations in patients with sepsis and infection. *Lancet.* 1993;341:515-518.

[29] Reinhart K, Meisner M. Biomarkers in the critically ill patient: procalcitonin. *Crit. Care Clin.* 2011;27:253-263.

[30] Shehabi Y, Seppelt I. Pro/con debate: is procalcitonin useful for guiding antibiotic decision making in critically ill patients? *Crit. Care.* 2008;12:211-6.

[31] Reinhart K, Karzai W, Meisner M. Procalcitonin as a systemic inflammatory response to infection. *Intensive Care Med.* 2000;26:1193-200.

[32] Müller B, Becker KL, Schächinger H, et al. Calcitonin precursors are reliable markers of sepsis in a medical intensive care unit. *Crit Care Med.* 2000;28(4):977–83.

[33] Selberg O, Hecker H, Martin M, et al. Discrimination of sepsis and systemic inflammatory response syndrome by determination of circulating plasma concentrations of procalcitonin, protein complement 3a, and interleukin-6. *Crit. Care Med.* 2000;28:2793–8.

[34] Castelli GP, Pognani C, Meisner M, et al. Procalcitonin and C-reactive protein during systemic inflammatory response syndrome, sepsis and organ dysfunction. *Crit. Care.* 2004;8:R234–40.

[35] Uzzan B, Cohen R, Nocholas P, et al. Procalcitonin as adiagnostic test for sepsis in critically ill adults and after surgery or trauma: a systematic review and metaanalysis. *Crit. Care Med.* 2006;34:1996-2003.

[36] Deis JN, Creech CB, Estrada CM, Abramo TJ. Procalcitonin as a marker of severe bacterial infection in children in the emergency department. *Pediatr. Emerg. Care.* 2010;26(1):51-63.

[37] Gilbert DN. Use of plasma procalcitonin levels as an adjuct to clinical microbiology. *J. Clin. Microbiol.* 2010;48(7):2325-2329.

[38] Ugarte H, Silva E, Mercan D, De Mendinca A, Vincent JL. Procalcitonin used as a marker of infection in the intensive care unit. *Crit. Care Med.* 1999;27(3):498-504.

[39] Sakr Y, Sponhoz C, Tuche F, Brunhorst F, Reinhart K. The role of procalcitonin in febrile neutropenic patients: review of the literature. *Infection.* 2008;36(5);396-407.

[40] Jensen JU, Hein L, Lundgren B, et al. Procalcitonin and survival study (PASS) group. Procalcitonin-guided interventions against infections to increase early appropriate antibiotics and improve survival in the intensive care unit: a randomized trial. *Crit care Med.* 2011;39(9):2048-2058.

[41] Reinhart K, Meisner M. Biomarkers in the critically ill patient: procalcitonin. *Crit Care Clin.* 2011;27:253-263.

[42] Schuetz P, Briel M, Christ-Crain M, et al. Procalcitonin to guide initiation and duration of antibiotic treatment in acute respiratory infections: an individual patient data meta-analysis. *Clin. Infect Dis.* 2012 Sep;55(5):651-62.

[43] Lopez AF, Cubells CL, Garcia JJG, Pou JF. Procalcitonin in pediatric emergency departments for the early diagnosis of invasive bacterial infections in febrile infants: results of a multicenter study and utility of a rapid qualitative test for this marker. *Pediatr. Infect Dis J.* 2003;22(10):895-903.

[44] Becker KL, Snider R, Nylen ES. Procalcitinin assay in systemic inflammation, infection and sepsis: clinical utility and limitations. *Crit. Care Med.* 2008;36(3):941-952.

[45] Tang BM, Eslick GD, Craig JC, et al. Accuracy of procalcitonin for sepsis diagnosis in critically ill patients: systematic review and meta-analysis. *Lancet Infect Dis.* 2007;7:210–7.

[46] Kibe S, Adams K, Barlow G. Diagnostic and prognostic biomarkers of sepsis in critical care. *J. Antimicrob Chemother.* 2011;66(2):ii33-ii40.

[47] Uusitalo-Seppälä R, Koskinen P, Leino A, Peuravuori H, Vahlberg T, Rintala EM. Early detectionof severe sepsis in the emergency room: diagnostic value of plasma C-reactive protein, procalcitonin, and interleukin-6. *Scand. J. Infect. Dis.* 2011;43(11-12),883–890.

[48] Bozza FA, Salluh JI, Japiassu AM, et al. Cytokine profiles as markers of disease severity in sepsis: a multiplex analysis. *Crit. Care.* 2007;11(2):R49.

[49] Oberholzer A, Souza SM, Tschoeke SK, et al. Plasma cytokine measurements augment prognostic scores as indicators of outcome in patients with severe sepsis. *Shock.* 2005;23(6): 488–493.

[50] Mera S, Tatulescu D, Cismaru C, et al. Multiplex cytokine profiling in patients with sepsis. *APMIS.* 2011; 119(2):155–163.

[51] Mehr S, Doyle LW. Cytokines as markers of bacterial sepsis in newborn infants: a review. *Pediatr Infect Dis J.* 2000 Sep;19(9):879-87.

[52] Smulian JC, Vintzileos AM, Lai YL, Santiago J, Shen-Schwarz S, Campbell WA. Maternal chorioamnionitis and umbilical vein interleukin-6 levels for identifying early neonatal sepsis. *J. Matern Fetal Med.* 1999 May-Jun;8(3):88-94.

[53] Franz AR, Steinbach G, Kron M, Pohlandt F. Interleukin-8: a valuable tool to restrict antibiotic therapy in newborn infants. *Acta Paediatr.* 2001 Sep;90(9):1025-32.

[54] Vincent JL, Beumier M. Diagnostic and prognostic markers in sepsis. *Expert Rev Anti Infect Ther.* 2013; 11(3):265-275.

[55] Bouchon A, Facchetti F, Weigand MA, Colonna M. TREM-1 amplifies inflammation and is a crucial mediator of septic shock. *Nature.* 2001;410(6832),1103-1107.

[56] Gibot S. Clinical review:role of triggering receptor expressed on myeloid cells-1 during sepsis. *Crit. Care.* 2005;9(5):485-489.

[57] Barraud D, Gibot S. Triggering receptor expressed on myeloid cell 1. *Crit care Clin.* 2011;27:265-279.

[58] Gibot S, Kolopp-Sarda MN, Bene MC, et al. Plasma level of a triggering receptor expressed on myeloid cells-1: its diagnostic accuracy in patients with suspected sepsis. *Ann Intern Med.* 2004;141(1):9-15.

[59] Zhang J, She D, Feng D, Jia Y, Xie L. Dynamic changes of serum soluble triggering receptor expressed on myeloid cells-1 (sTREM-1) reflect sepsis severity and can predict prognosis: a prospective study. *BMC Infect. Dis.* 2011;11:53.

[60] Barati M, Bashar FR, Shahrami R, et al. Soluble triggering receptor expressed on myeloid cells 1 and the diagnosis of sepsis. *J. Crit Care.* 2010;25(2):362, e1–6.

[61] Gamez-Diaz LY, Enriquez LE, Mature JD, et al. Diagnostic accuracy of HMGB-1, sTREM-1, and CD64 as markers of sepsis in patients recently admitted to the emergency department. *Acad. Emerg. Med.*2011;18(8):807-815.

[62] Swarnkar K, Vagha J. Sepsis biomarkers in early onset neonatal infections: a review. *The Internet Journal of Infectious Diseases.* 2013; 11(1).

[63] Cid J, García-Pardo G, Aguinaco R, Sánchez R, Llorente A. Neutrophil CD64: diagnostic accuracy and prognostic value in patients presenting to the emergency department. *Eur. J. Clin. Microbiol. Infect. Dis.*2011;30(7):845–852.

[64] Gros A, Roussel M, Sauvadet E, et al. The sensitivity of neutrophil CD64 expression as a biomarker of bacterial infection is low in critically ill patients. *Intensive Care Med.* 2012;38(3):445–452).

[65] Cetinkaya M, Ozkan H, Koksal N, Celebi S, Hacimustafaoglu M. Comparison of serum amyloid A concentrations with those of C-reactive protein and procalcitonin in diagnosis and follow-up of neonatal sepsis in premature infants. *J. Perinatol.* 2009;29(3):225-231.

[66] Arnon S, Litmanovitz I. Diagnostic tests in neonatal sepsis. *Curr. Opin. Infect Dis.* 2008;21:223-227.

[67] Yuan H, Huang J, Lv B, et al. Diagnosis value of the serum amyloid A test in neonatal sepsis: a meta-analysis. *BioMed Research International.* 2013; 520294.

[68] LaRosa SP., Opal SM. Biomarkers: the future. *Crit Care Clin.* 2011;27:407-419.

[69] Opal SM, Scannon PJ, Vincent JL, et al. Relationship between plasma levels of lipopolysacharide (LPS) and LPS-binding protein in patients with severe sepsis and sepstic shock. *J. Infect Dis.* 1999;180:1584-9.

[70] Marshall JC, Walker PM, Foster DM, et al. *Crit Care.* 2002Aug;6(4):342-8.

[71] Siner JM, Bhandari V, Engle KM, Elias JA, Siegel MD. Elevated serum angiopoietin 2 levels are associated with increased mortality in sepsis. *Shock.* 2009 Apr;31(4):348-53.

[72] Ricciuto DR, dos Santos CC, Hawkes M, et al. Angiopoietin-1 and angiopoietin-2 as clinically informative prognostic biomarkers of morbidity and mortality in severe sepsis. *Crit. Care Med.* 2011;39(4):702-710.

[73] Gibot S, Massin F, Cravoisy A, et al. Growth arrest-specific protein 6 plasma concentrations during septic shock. *Crit Care.* 2007;11(1)R8.

[74] Borgel D, Clauser S, Bornstain C, et al. Elevated growth-arrest-specific protein 6 plasma levels in patients with severe sepsis. *Crit Care Med.* 2006 Jan;34(1):219-22.

[75] Dark PM, Dean P, Warhurst G. Bench-to-bedside review: the promise of rapid infection diagnosis during sepsis using polymerase chain reaction-based pathogen detection. *Crit Care*. 2009;13(4):217.

[76] Pasqualini L, Mencacci A, Leli C, et al. Diagnostic performance of a multiple real-time PCR assay in patients with suspected sepsis hospitalized in an internal medicine ward. *J. Clin Microbiol*. 2012;50(4):1285-1288.

[77] Fitting C, Parlato M, Adib-Conquy M, et al. DNAemia detection by multiplex PCR and biomarkers for infection in systemic inflammatory response syndrome patients. *PLoS ONE*. 2012;7(6), e38916.

In: Sepsis
Editor: Nancy Khardori

ISBN: 978-1-63117-244-1

Chapter 9

Intricacies of Hyperglycemia and Disordered Glucose Metabolism in Sepsis

Jagdeesh Ullal, M.D., Valeria Bohrt-Terceros, M.D., and Romesh Khardori, M.D., Ph.D.
Division of Endocrinology and Metabolism,
Department of Internal Medicine,
Eastern Virginia Medical School,
Norfolk, VA, US

Abstract

Hyperglycemia often develops in the absence of diabetes mellitus (stress hyperglycemia) and its prevalence in sepsis remains high. In the backdrop of pre-existing diabetes, rapid metabolic decompensation ensues when patients become septic. Hyperglycemia is associated with oxidative / inflammatory stress that has the potential to compound sepsis induced cytokine mediated tissue injury. This construct has been basis for implementing intensified glucose control protocols during management of people with critical illness/sepsis. Recently questions have been raised about the validity of need for intensified strict glycemic control in critical illness including sepsis.

Based on review of clinical trials and position statements from professional societies, we have reviewed mechanisms of dysglycemia and recommended glucose targets to guide readers in managing patients with sepsis effectively while avoiding hypoglycemia at the same time. Plasma glucose target of 140 -180 mg/dl appears to be safe and effective for most patients. This can effectively be achieved by intravenous infusion of insulin that is amenable to rapid correction to avoid unintended hypoglycemia. More and more hospitals are using computerized insulin titration protocols that reduce the likelihood of inducing hypoglycemia that is now considered a serious threat to survival.

Introduction

Hyperglycemia goes hand in hand with physiologic stress and this phenomenon is in part an evolutionary mechanism to ensure that the central nervous system has nutrients to function in the time of crisis. Hyperglycemia often develops in the absence of diabetes mellitus (stress hyperglycemia) and its prevalence in sepsis is high [1]. Alternatively hyperglycemia may represent previously undiagnosed diabetes mellitus or stress induced exacerbation of hyperglycemia in a patient with known diabetes mellitus. Hyperglycemia has been seen in patients with critical illness such as acute coronary syndromes (ACS) or stroke. This has sparked great debate in utility versus futility of strict glycemic control and clinical outcomes. This debate is far from settled and evidence seems to favor less stringent control. Recent Cochrane review found no evidence of better outcome with strict glycemic control when insulin was used to treat patients with acute ischemic stroke [2]. However, this extrapolation to sepsis cannot always be made since ACS and stroke syndromes are organ specific problem whereas, sepsis is a multisystem involvement with significantly wider ramifications.

Sepsis is a clinical syndrome that is a complication of severe infection and is characterized by systemic inflammation and widespread tissue injury. This is a microbial phenomenon in which an inflammatory response to the presence of microorganisms or the invasion of normally sterile host tissue by these organisms is characteristic. Given this systemic inflammatory response and that acute hyperglycemia induces an increase in inflammatory cytokines like plasma IL-6, TNF-α, and IL-18 concentrations[3], questions still remain as to whether this hyperglycemic response in sepsis is protective or detrimental and whether this additional oxidative and inflammatory stress is only adding fuel to fire in the context of sepsis. In this review we examine the role of hyperglycemia, the pathophysiologic mechanisms of hyperglycemia in sepsis, additional consequences of hyperglycemia, and therapeutic options.

Endotoxemia, Inflammation and Insulin Resistance

Dysglycemia/Hyperglycemia in acute setting of an inflammatory state are suggestive of insulin resistance. Insulin resistance and inflammation are intimately linked [4]. It is shown that inflammatory mediators absorbed through the gut, such as lipopolysaccharide (LPS), may cause chronic subclinical inflammation. Endotoxemia occurs when LPS (endotoxin) reaches the circulatory system [5]. LPS can induce an immune response, activating pathways that cause inflammation, which in turn inhibits insulin signaling.

Insulin resistance is characterized by the activation of two important inflammatory pathways namely the NF-kappaB and the c-Jun NH2-terminal kinase (JNK) pathway [6]. These pathways are activated by many of the same pro-inflammatory stimuli including cytokines such as TNF, and the involvement of toll-like receptors. The toll-like receptors can be triggered by bacterial, viral or fungal pathogens and also by fatty acids [7]. TLR4 is the receptor for LPS and plays a critical role in innate immunity. Following binding of LPS to TLR4 and its co-receptors - CD14 and MD-2, adaptor protein myeloid differentiation factor 88 (MyD88) is recruited to the Toll/IL-1 receptor (TIR) domain of the receptor. Interaction of the TIR domain of TLR4 and MyD88 triggers a downstream signaling cascade involving activation of the NF-kappaB pathway, which in turn activates the transcription of many pro-inflammatory genes encoding cytokines, chemokines, and other effectors of the innate immune response [8]. These inflammatory kinases may promote insulin resistance by down-regulating components of the insulin signaling cascade.

Immune Dysfunction in Hyperglycemia

Acute, short-term hyperglycemia affects major components of innate immunity and impairs the ability of the host to combat infection with distinctive pro-inflammatory alterations of the immune response. Tissue damage caused by injury or by invading pathogenic microorganisms choreographs a complex of inflammatory response with ultimate aim of lysis or phagocytosis of invading organisms and restoration of physiologic conditions. The onset of hyperglycemia in previously non diabetic patients possibly can be ascribed to increased stress hormone release compounding peripheral insulin resistance, drugs that impair insulin action or secretion like (steroids and catecholamines), and excessive dextrose administration.

Role of Cortisol on Hyperglycemia in Sepsis

Cortisol plays a vital supportive role in the maintenance of vascular tone, endothelial integrity, and vascular permeability that in turn affect distribution of total body water within the vascular compartment. Its secretion is governed by the integrity of hypothalamo-pitutiary adrenal axis. Other factors such as endothelin and atrial natriuretic hormone may also play role in elevation of cortisol thus accounting for dissociation between plasma cortisol and adrencorticotropin (ACTH) levels in critically ill patients [9]. Cortisol potentiates the vasoconstrictor actions of catecholamines. There is a significant drop in cortisol binding globulin (CBG) in sepsis and this is reflected as a higher free cortisol level. Following this there is an increase and normalization of CBG levels, independent from clinical parameters from the initial onset of septic shock indicating that CBG plays an active role in the glucocorticoid response to severe stress and in the regulation of cortisol availability to target tissues [10]. Most laboratory assays measure bound cortisol and the results can be erroneous in the context of sepsis. Measurement of free cortisol would be preferable.

The Surviving Sepsis Campaign, an international effort to increase awareness and improve outcome in severe sepsis, recommended treatment with corticosteroids like hydrocortisone with or without the addition of fludrocortisone in patients with septic shock who, despite adequate fluid replacement, require vasopressor therapy to maintain adequate blood pressure [11]. Since glucocorticoids stimulate gluconeogenesis, treatment with steroids may be accompanied by hyperglycemia and therefore increased need for using insulin [12,13]. It has been suggested that continuous infusion of glucocorticoids rather than boluses results in better glycemic control [14].

Glycemic Targets in Sepsis

A protocol driven approach to insulin therapy for management of hyperglycemia above 180 mg/dl has been recommended by the 2012 Surviving Sepsis Campaign Committee [15]. Close monitoring (every 1-2 hours) is recommended because of a relatively narrow range for blood glucose targets. Several medical societies including American Association of Clinical Endocrinologists, American Diabetes Association, American College of Physicians, and Society of Critical Care Medicine seem to endorse this position [16-18]. These societies endorse glucose target between 140 and 180 mg/dL. There is no evidence that targets between 140 and 180 mg/dL are significantly different from targets of 110 to 140 mg/dL [19], and this level is recommended for all patient with hyperglycemia regardless of a previous history of disordered glucose metabolism.

The need for revision of glycemic targets in critically sick patients arose out of concerns for real impact on clinical outcome and the safety. This was after the initial euphoria from Van den Berghe's trial in surgical intensive care unit (SICU), where patients that had spent 5 or more days in the SICU, showed a dramatic reduction of episodes of septicemia by 46 % when blood glucose was targeted between 80-110 mgs/dl [20]. In this study patients were classified post-hoc to severe sepsis.

The first trial that specifically evaluated effect of intensified glucose control in patients with severe sepsis was the VISEP trial conducted across 18 academic centers in Germany [21]. This study failed to show any beneficial effect from intensive glucose control, and instead revealed significantly increased risk for severe hypoglycemia. No survival benefit was shown either. Another study where both corticosteroids and intensive insulin therapy were used together in patients with septic shock (COIITSS) [included 509 patients with septic shock randomly assigned in 11 intensive care units in France], again no advantage was seen. On the contrary patients experienced more episodes of hypoglycemia and there was non-significant increase in risk of dearth [22].

At the present preponderance of evidence leads to infer that intensive glucose control, in critically sick patients or in those with severe sepsis, does not reduce length of hospital stay or mortality. In an elegant focused review, controversies surrounding management of critically ill patients with severe sepsis have been discussed by Simon Finfer [23]. To date the largest study to evaluate effects of intensive glucose control in critically ill patients is the "Normoglycemia in Intensive Care Evaluation Survival Using Glucose Algorithm Regulation (NICE-SUGAR)". This study was undertaken in Australia, New Zealand, Canada and the Unites states. In this study, 6104 patients underwent randomization to a blood glucose target of either 81-108 mg/dL, or < 180 mgs/dL. Eight hundred and twenty nine patients in the intensive treatment group (27.5%) and 751 in the control group (24.9%) died. Thus, the odds of dying with intensive control were 1.14 times greater than with conventional control (p=0.02) [24]. Across all type of critically ill patients, the NICE-SUGAR revealed that targeting blood glucose less than <108 mg/dl with insulin increased 90 day mortality from 24.9 to 27.5% as compared with the glucose target of 140–180 mg/dl. Excess deaths were attributed to cardiovascular causes although the cause remains unclear as to the triggers. In this trial patients with sepsis at baseline were identified as a predefined subgroup. There was no evidence that patient with severe sepsis any differently from non-septic critically sick patients.

Management of Hyperglycemia in Sepsis

Management of severe sepsis consists of antibiotics, use of supportive therapies to sustain life while waiting for the adverse effects of sepsis-induced organ dysfunction to abate. Central role of supportive therapies cannot be overemphasized.

The Surviving Sepsis Campaign published in 2010 included glucose control maintained over lower limit of normal but less than 150mg/dl, as part of their "Sepsis Management Bundle" to be accomplished over the first 24 hours [25]. The use of a multifaceted performance improvement initiative was successful in changing sepsis treatment behavior as reflected in significant increase in compliance with sepsis performance measures.

Insulin is the most effective agent for management of hyperglycemia in the majority of hospitalized patients. Intravenous insulin infusion is the most preferred route. A close monitoring of blood glucose (1-2 hourly) allows for rapid corrections and, therefore, avoidance of wide fluctuations in blood glucose. The threshold to start insulin treatment is blood glucose of ≤180 mg/dL. Once insulin infusion is started, the blood glucose should be maintained between 140 and 180 mg/dL; a lower BG target (110–140 mg/dL) may be appropriate in selected patients. Targets of <110 mg/dL or >180 mg/dL are no longer recommended [26]. This conclusion is reinforced by recent reviews, meta-analysis of randomized controlled trials and the most recent Clinical Practice Guidelines of Canadian Diabetes Association [27-29].

Glycemic control is achieved safely and effectively with an intravenous insulin protocol implemented by staff or, most recently, by a computerized system. Computerized insulin titration protocol improves glucose control by increasing the percentage of glucose values in range, reducing hyperglycemia, and reducing severe hypoglycemia [30].

Conclusion

Management of hyperglycemia in patients with sepsis has been subject several observational and controlled studies. Initial enthusiasm to enforce tighter glycemic control has been supplanted by more nuanced approach primarily focusing on targets that are safe and relatively free from increasing any harm to the patients. Hypoglycemia remains a serious limitation to achieve tighter glycemic control even within the ranges currently accepted by the clinicians. Newer tools of insulin delivery and closer surveillance significantly reduce the burden of hypoglycemia. There is no convincing evidence that Blood Glucose levels of less than 140 mgs/dL ensure better outcome including lessening of the risk of death.

References

[1] Rattanataweeboon, P; Vilaichone, W; Vannasaeng, S. Stress hyperglycemia in patients with sepsis. *J Med Assoc Thai*, 2009, 92 Suppl 2, S88-S94.

[2] Bellolio, MF; Gilmore, RM; Stead, LG. Insulin for glycaemic control in acute ischaemic stroke (Review). *Cochrane Diabetes Syst Rev*, 2011, (9), CD005346.

[3] Esposito, K; Nappo, F; Marfella, R; Giugliano, G; Giugliano, F; Ciotola, M; Quagliaro, L; Ceriello, A; Giugliano, D. Inflammatory cytokine concentrations are acutely increased by hyperglycemia in humans, role of oxidative stress. *Circulation*, 106, 2067-2072, 2002.

[4] Shoelson, SE; Lee, J; Goldfine, AB. Inflammation and insulin resistance. *J Clin Invest*, 116, 1793-1801, 2006.

[5] Ding, S; Chi, MM; Scull, BP; Rigby, R; Schwerbrock, NM; Magness, S; Jobin, C; Lund, PK. High-fat diet: bacteria interactions promote intestinal inflammation which precedes and correlates with obesity and insulin resistance in mouse. *PLoS One*, 5, e12191, 2010.

[6] Andreasen, AS; Kelly, M; Berg, RM; Moller, K; Pedersen, BK. Type 2 diabetes is associated with altered NF-kappaB DNA binding activity, JNK phosphorylation, and AMPK phosphorylation in skeletal muscle after LPS. *PLoS One*, 6, e23999, 2011.

[7] Shi, H; Kokoeva, MV; Inouye, K; Tzameli, I; Yin, H; Flier, JS. TLR4 links innate immunity and fatty acid-induced insulin resistance. *J Clin Invest*, 116, 3015-3025, 2006.

[8] Siebler, J; Galle, PR; Weber, MM. The gut-liver-axis: endotoxemia, inflammation, insulin resistance and NASH. *J Hepatol*, 48, 1032-1034, 2008.

[9] Vermes, I; Beishuizen, A; Hampsink, RM; Haanen, C. Dissociation of plasma adrenocorticotropin and cortisol levels in critically ill patients, possible role of endothelin and atrial natriuretic hormone. *J Clin Endocrinol Metab*, 80, 1238-1242, 1995.

[10] Beishuizen, A; Thijs, LG; Vermes, I. Patterns of corticosteroid-binding globulin and the free cortisol index during septic shock and multitrauma. *Intensive Care Med*, 27, 1584-1591, 2001.

[11] Dellinger, RP; Carlet, JM; Masur, H; Gerlach, H; Calandra, T; Cohen, J; Gea-Banacloche, J; Keh, D; Marshall, JC; Parker, MM; Ramsay, G; Zimmerman, JL; Vincent, JL; Levy, MM. Surviving Sepsis Campaign guidelines for management of severe sepsis and septic shock. *Intensive Care Med*, 30, 536-555, 2004.

[12] Khani, S; Tayek, JA. Cortisol increases gluconeogenesis in humans: its role in the metabolic syndrome. *Clin Sci (Lond)*, 101, 739-747, 2001.

[13] Rady, MY; Johnson, DJ; Patel, BM; Larson, JS; Helmers, RA. Influence of individual characteristics on outcome of glycemic control in intensive care unit patients with or without diabetes mellitus. *Mayo Clin Proc*, 80, 1558-1567, 2005.

[14] Loisa, P; Parviainen, I; Tenhunen, J; Hovilehto, S; Ruokonen, E. Effect of mode of hydrocortisone administration on glycemic control in patients with septic shock: a prospective randomized trial. *Crit Care*, 11, R21, 2007.

[15] Dellinger, RP; Levy, MM; Rhodes, A; Annane, D; Gerlach, H; Opal, SM; Sevransky, JE; Sprung, CL; Douglas, IS; Jaeschke, R; Osborn, TM; Nunnally, ME; Townsend, SR; Reinhart, K; Kleinpell, RM; Angus, DC; Deutschman, CS; Machado, FR; Rubenfeld, GD; Webb, S; Beale, RJ; Vincent, JL; Moreno, R. Surviving Sepsis Campaign: international guidelines for management of severe sepsis and septic shock, 2012. *Intensive Care Med*, 39, 165-228, 2013.

[16] Moghissi, ES; Korytkowski, MT; DiNardo, M; Einhorn, D; Hellman, R; Hirsch, IB; Inzucchi, SE; Ismail-Beigi, F; Kirkman, MS; Umpierrez, GE. American Association of

Clinical Endocrinologists and American Diabetes Association consensus statement on inpatient glycemic control. *Endocr Pract*, 15, 353-369, 2009.

[17] Qaseem, A; Chou, R; Humphrey, LL; Shekelle, P., Inpatient Glycemic Control: Best Practice Advice From the Clinical Guidelines Committee of the American College of Physicians. *Am J Med Qual*, 2013.

[18] Jacobi, J; Bircher, N; Krinsley, J; Agus, M; Braithwaite, SS; Deutschman, C; Freire, AX; Geehan, D; Kohl, B; Nasraway, SA; Rigby, M; Sands, K; Schallom, L; Taylor, B; Umpierrez, G; Mazuski, J; Schunemann, H., Guidelines for the use of an insulin infusion for the management of hyperglycemia in critically ill patients. *Crit Care Med*, 40, 3251-3276, 2012.

[19] Standards of medical care in diabetes--2012. *Diabetes Care*, 35 Suppl, 1, S11-S63, 2012.

[20] van den Berghe, G; Wouters, P; Weekers, F; Verwaest, C; et al. Intensive insulin therapy in critically ill patients. *N Engl J Med*, 345, 1359-1367, 2001

[21] Brunkhorst, FM; Engel, C; Bloos, F; Meier-Hellmann, A; Ragaller, M; Weiler, N; Moerer, O; Gruendling, M; Oppert, M; Grond, S; Olthoff, D; Jaschinski, U; John, S; Rossaint, R; Welte, T; Schaefer, M; Kern, P; Kuhnt, E; Kiehntopf, M; Hartog, C; Natanson, C; Loeffler, M; Reinhart, K., Intensive insulin therapy and pentastarch resuscitation in severe sepsis. *N Engl J Med*, 358, 125-139, 2008.

[22] Annane, D; Cariou, A; Maxime, V; Azoulay, E, et al. COIITSS Study Investigators. Corticosteroid treatment and intensive insulin therapy for septic shock in adults: a randomized controlled trial. *JAMA*, 303, 341-348, 2010.

[23] Finfer, S, Clinical controversies in the management of critically ill patients with severe sepsis: Resuscitation fluids and glucose control. *Virulence*, 4, 2013.

[24] NICE-SUGAR Study Investigators. Intensive versus conventional glucose control in critically ill patients. *N Engl J Med*, 360, 1283-1297, 2009.

[25] Levy, MM; Dellinger, RP; Townsend, SR; Linde-Zwirble, WT; et al. The Surviving Sepsis Campaign: results of an international guideline-based performance improvement program targeting severe sepsis. *Intensive Care Med*, 36, 222-231, 2010.

[26] Moghissi, ES. Reexamining the evidence for inpatient glucose control, new recommendations for glycemic targets. *Am J Health Syst Pharm*, 67, S3-S8, 2010.

[27] Ling, Y; Li, X, and, Gao, X. Intetnsive versus conventional glucose control in critically ill patients: A meta-analysis of randomized controlled trials. *Eur J Intern Med*, 23, 564-574, 2012.

[28] Kuppinger, D; and, Hartl, WH. In search of the perfect glucose concentration for hospitalized patients, A brief review of meta-analysis. *Nutrition*, 29, 708-712, 2013.

[29] Canadian Diabetes Association Clinical Practice Guidelines Expert Committee. In-hospital Management od Diabetes. *Can J Med*, 37, S77-S81, 2013.

[30] Klonoff, DC. Intensive insulin therapy in critically ill hospitalized patients, making it safe and effective. *J Diabetes Sci Technol*, 5, 755-767, 2011.

Index

A

D

E

F

G

H

I

J

K

L

M

N

O

P

Q

R

S

T

U

V

W

Y